KINESIOLOGY OF EXERCISE

KINESIOLOGY OF EXERCISE

A Safe and Effective Way to Improve
Athletic Performance

Michael Yessis, Ph.D.

MP

MASTERS PRESS

A Subsidiary of Howard W. Sams & Co.

Published by Masters Press
(A Division of Howard W. Sams & Co.)
2647 Waterfront Parkway East Drive
Suite 300
Indianapolis, IN 46214

All rights reserved. Published 1993
First printing, February 1992
Fifth printing, May 1994

Printed in the United States of America.

Library of Congress Cataloging-in-Publication Data

Yessis, Michael.
     Kinesiology of exercise: a safe and effective way to improve athletic performance / Michael Yessis.
          p. cm.
     ISBN: 0-940279-36-3: $17.95
     1. Kinesiology.   2. Weight lifting -- Physiological aspects.
   I. Title
QP303.Y47 1992   92-1211
613.7'13--dc20   CIP

CONTENTS

PART ONE   THE LOWER BODY

Chapter 1   The Ankle   3

Chapter 2   The Knee Joint   11

Chapter 3   The Hip Joint and Pelvic Girdle   19

Chapter 4   Combination Exercises   37

ACKNOWLEDGMENTS

I would like to express my thanks to the following people:

- Mr. Joe Weider, for giving me the opportunity to write about exercises in *Muscle and Fitness* magazine.
- To my many readers, who kept asking me for a book of this nature.
- To Larry McDaniel, for his patience and expertise in taking the photographs for this book.
- To Tom Yessis, who worked so diligently on producing the great artwork.
- To models Paula Piwarunas, Joe Ward, Bill Evans, and others, who all worked many long hours performing all the exercises.
- To Cecilia Tobin and Jackie Ehrman, for their extensive typing of the manuscript.
- To my wife, Edie, for her suggestions and support.
- To my daughter, Marissa, for keeping me laughing.

INTRODUCTION

The term *kinesiology* has become popular in fitness and sports training literature. The reason for this is simple, because kinesiology is the science of movement. Through kinesiology, the movements taking place in an exercise or sports movement and the muscles involved can more accurately be described. In addition, through the science of kinesiology, it is possible to determine the type of muscular contraction involved in an exercise and how the muscular involvement changes with different positions, grips, and techniques.

Kinesiology of Exercise contains easy-to-read, detailed explanations of the free weight and machine strength exercises for bodybuilding and many different sports. Included are explanations of how you should execute each exercise safely and effectively, how different muscles are involved, and the changes that take place when changes in technique are made. Also included is information about which sports or sports movements duplicate or are similar to the actions and muscles involved in each exercise.

This book also contains basic information about the biomechanics of exercise. In biomechanics, the principles of mechanics are applied to an exercise to determine how it should be done for maximum safety and effectiveness. Included are factors such as momentum, acceleration, force, inertia, levers, and angle of muscle pull.

By using the key kinesiological and biomechanical concepts, I have developed a comprehensive text of basic strength exercises. By carefully reading this book and referring to it as you exercise, you will learn the best way to do the exercises for the effects you desire. In some cases because of the amount and the "newness" of much of the information, I strongly recommend reading the exercises more than once. As a result you will know exactly which muscles are involved in the exercise, depending upon your grip, the equipment, and your method of execution.

You will also learn the many factors that are involved in making each exercise maximally safe and effective. In some cases, you can learn how to do the exercise even if you have a particular physical problem. For example, you will find out how you can tax the muscles in the same manner with light weights as you can with heavy weights but without the same stress on the spine.

By performing the exercises in this book and closely following the guidelines for execution, you can increase your body's muscular development. Athletes will notice a distinct improvement in their sports performance. It is important to understand that strength, especially of the specific muscles involved, is the basis for speed, coordination, agility, and even flexibility. Without adequate levels of strength, you will never be able to achieve your maximum performances. In addition, adequate levels of strength are the key to the prevention of injury, not only in sports, but at your job and at home as well.

PART ONE

The Lower Body

1 The Ankle

ANATOMY OF THE ANKLE

The ankle is formed by the junction of three bones: the talus bone of the foot and the tibia and fibula bones of the shin. The ligaments that tie and hold the ankle joint together limit the joint's voluntary movement to about 60 degrees. However, if the body's weight and external weights are used, the range of motion of the ankle can be increased.

BASIC MOVEMENTS IN THE ANKLE

Only two movements are possible in the ankle joint. The first is flexion, also known as dorsi flexion, or the movement of the toes (foot) toward the shin. The second is extension, also known as plantar flexion, or the movement of the toes (foot) away from the body. When you are in contact with the floor, ankle joint extension raises your body, and when you are airborne, it points your toes.

There are two additional movements of the foot that are not true ankle joint movements. They are inversion and eversion, which take place between the talus (ankle bone) and the navicular (tarsal bone) and the calcaneus (heel bone). This joint is known as the subtalar joint.

In inversion, also known as adduction or supination, the sole of the foot is turned inward and upward. In eversion, also known as abduction or pronation, the sole of the foot is turned outward and upward, that is, the toe area of the foot is pointed outward. These movements are an important part of the pushing-off actions required by athletes in many sports. Development of the muscles involved in eversion and inversion helps prevent ankle sprains.

MAJOR MUSCLES INVOLVED

The muscles of the ankle and foot have a very intricate structure. There are muscles that affect only the toes, others that affect the toes and the ankle, and still others that work only the ankle and, in some cases, the ankle and the knee. Many of these muscles have more than one action, so in order to have only one movement it is necessary to have other muscles participate to prevent secondary actions.

In dorsi flexion (raising the foot toward the shin), which occurs in the toe raise exercise, the tibialis anterior, extensor digitorum longus, and peroneus tertius muscles are involved (see Figure 1.1). The tibialis anterior is a long, slender muscle situated on the front of the shin. It originates at the upper surface of the tibia (the major bone of the shin) and inserts on the underside of the medial cuneiform bone of the foot (almost in the middle of the foot). The tibialis anterior is also involved in inversion. It works together with the tibialis posterior, which is located deep beneath the calf muscles.

The extensor digitorum longus is similar to the tibialis anterior and lies next to it on its outside edge. The extensor digitorum longus originates on the condyle of the tibia and the

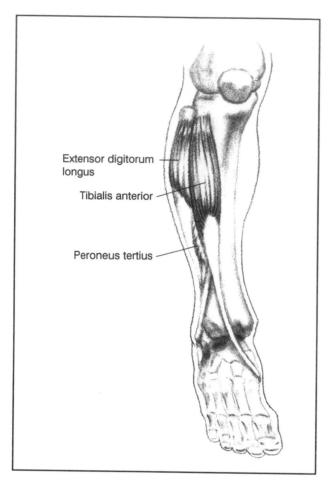

Figure 1.1
Anterior view of the lower leg

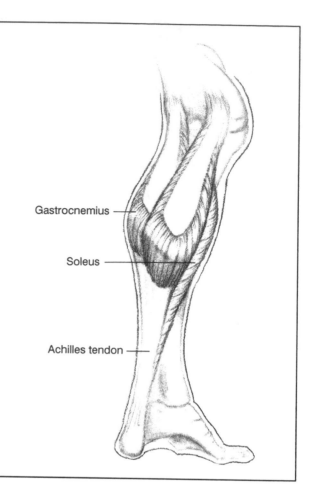

Figure 1.2
Side-posterior view of the lower leg

upper three-fourths of the fibula and inserts on the upper side of the four lesser toes.

The peroneus tertius is a small muscle. It originates on the lower two-thirds of the fibula and inserts on the near end of the fifth metatarsal bone (middle to front of the foot).

In the heel raise and seated calf raise exercises, the major muscles of the posterior shin are involved (see Figures 1.2 and 1.3). They are the gastrocnemius, which shapes the back surface of the shin, and the soleus, which is slightly wider than the gastrocnemius and lies directly underneath it. Collectively, these muscles are known as the calf muscles or the triceps surae group.

The gastrocnemius has two distinct heads which lie side by side and can easily be seen if the muscle is well developed. Both heads origi-

nate by separate tendons from the condyles of the femur (thigh bone).

The soleus originates on the upper part of the posterior surfaces of the tibia and fibula. At the lower end these muscles combine into the Achilles tendon, which attaches to the calcaneus (heel bone). It should also be noted that at the knee joint the gastrocnemius is involved in knee joint flexion.

ANKLE EXERCISES

■ Heel Raise (Calf Raise)

The heel raise exercise, when done through a full range of motion, is one of the most effective

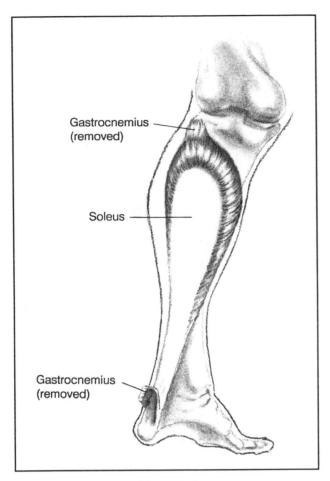

Figure 1.3
Side-posterior view of lower leg

leyball and basketball, height in diving, the push-off in the swimming start, and in trampolining. It is used in many other sports that require a combination of running and jumping, or for standing on the ball of the foot as in ballet. In bodybuilding the heel raise is very important for increasing bulk and for definition of the sides and upper back of the shins.

Execution

For greatest convenience, heel raises are done on an exercise machine. To do the exercise, place the balls of your feet on the raised platform and your shoulders under the resistance lever pads. On most machines the pads are lower than your shoulders, so you must squat to position yourself under the pads. As you do this, be sure to flex your knees and keep your spine erect at all times. Straighten your legs to assume the standing ready position. In this position, balance does not play a role. However, because of the importance of balance for athletes, as well as body-

and important exercises for almost all athletes and fitness buffs. Because of this, it belongs in almost everyone's arsenal of exercises.

Major muscles and actions involved

In the heel raise the gastrocnemius and soleus muscles of the shin are involved in plantar flexion (extension), as shown in Figure 1.4. In this action the heel is raised while the ball of the foot remains in contact with the platform. This action raises the entire body.

Sports uses

Ankle joint extension is a key action in all walking, running, and jumping activities. It provides the final push in propelling the body forward and upward as needed in race walking, speed running, high jumping, and long jumping. It is also used in jumping for a spike in volleyball, the jump shot in basketball, the block in vol-

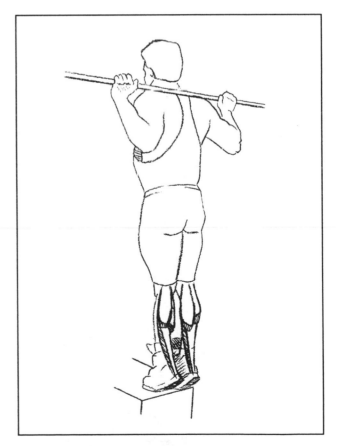

Figure 1.4
Muscles used in the heel raise

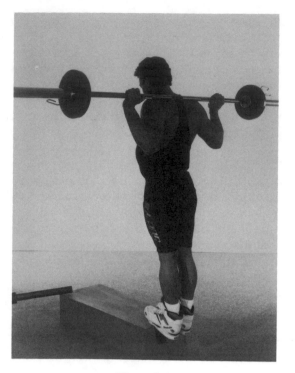

Photo 1.1

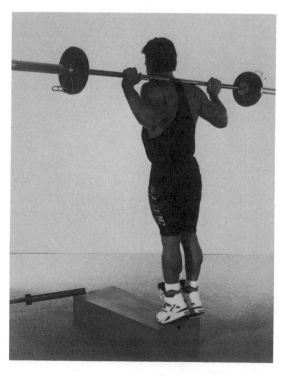

Photo 1.2

builders, execution of the heel raise in a free-standing position will be described.

To begin, place a barbell on the back of your shoulders or a dumbbell in each hand. Step up onto a beam or platform that is well secured and will not tip over. Place the balls of your feet on the edge of the platform with your feet hip- or shoulder-width apart. Point you toes forward.

When you are ready, inhale and hold your breath as you lower your heels until you feel a stretch in the Achilles tendon and calf muscles (see Photo 1.1). Hold your breath and with your spine held firmly, rise up as high as possible (see Photo 1.2). In the ending position, your heels should be raised maximally and your legs should be straight. Exhale and lower your body under control to the initial position. Pause momentarily to steady your balance and repeat.

Comments

• If you find that it is too difficult to go through the maximum range, use less resistance so that you can go as high and as low as possible. For most effective muscle development, it is very important to have full range of motion.

   If you are still unable to rise up high enough, most likely you have tight tendons and muscles. Thus, to increase the range of motion, you should do various ankle stretching exercises. This includes: 1) leaning into a wall with your feet 1–2 feet away from the wall and with your heels on the floor, and 2) doing full-range squats with no weight and with your heels on the floor at all times.

• To develop some of the assisting muscles and to bring in some other foot actions, you should change foot positions. For example, point your toes inward and then rise up. This positioning forces some inversion and development of the tibialis posterior (along with the muscles used in ankle joint extension). Pointing the toes outward and then doing heel raises uses foot eversion and the muscles involved (the three peroneal and extensor digitorum longus muscles located on the lateral sides of the lower legs). Placing the feet wider or narrower also changes the stress on the muscles and gives more all-around development.

• The gastrocnemius muscle is best developed when heel raises are done with the legs kept straight. In this position the muscle pulls very effectively in almost a straight line. However, if the knees are bent slightly, the gastrocnemius is less involved and greater stress falls on the soleus.

- The gastrocnemius is a two-joint muscle, crossing both the ankle and knee joints. Therefore, for maximum development it should be worked from both ends. Thus, to involve the gastrocnemius most effectively at the knee joint, knee curls or glute-ham-gastroc raises should be done.

- To do explosive type heel raises, use the muscle rebound effect. Assume the neutral foot position on a calf machine with the balls of your feet on the foot plate. When you are ready, inhale slightly more than usual and hold your breath as you lower your heels at a moderate rate of speed. Quickly reverse the position as soon as you feel a strong stretch on the Achilles tendon. The more you can lower your heels before reversing your direction, the more effective the exercise is in regard to sports specificity. Exhale and pause momentarily as you assume the neutral position before once again repeating the exercise.

- A variant of the heel raise is the donkey calf raise. To perform this exercise, assume a standing position and bend over from the hips so that your trunk is at a 90-degree angle to your legs. Have a partner sit on your hips as far back as possible for the resistance. Keep your legs straight and execute as you would heel raises. The donkey calf raise is an excellent substitute for the exercise machine heel raise. However, because body weight is used, the resistance is difficult to regulate. Only a donkey calf raise machine allows you to regulate the resistance.

■ Toe Raise

One of the most neglected parts of the body is the front of the shin. Part of the reason for this is that the muscles in this area do not have great mass and do very little in normal, everyday activities or in sports. However, this does not mean that they should be ignored. The shin muscles are most important in preventing injuries such as shin splints, and they also help to balance the development of the gastrocnemius and soleus to help prevent injury.

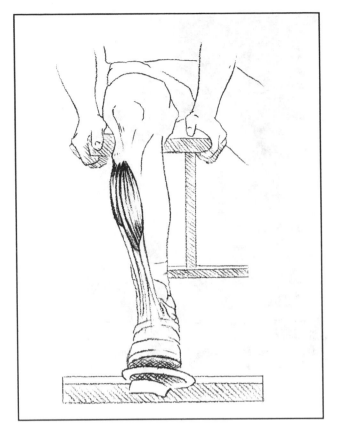

Figure 1.5
Muscles used in the toe raise

Major muscles and actions involved

Toe raises involve the tibialis anterior, extensor digitorum longus, and peroneus tertius muscles, all of which are located on the front of the shin (see Figure 1.5). These muscles are responsible for dorsi flexion.

Sports uses

The movement involved in dorsi flexion is very valuable in certain sports such as swimming (the breast stroke), cycling (the up phase), and running (to prepare for a touchdown). In walking and jogging dorsi flexion raises the toe area of the foot so it clears the ground during the swing phase. Its greatest value is in keeping the lower leg muscles in balance and for developing the lower legs of bodybuilders.

Execution

Variant 1: Sit on the edge of a bench or chair with your lower leg hanging straight down and with your heel on a raised platform. Place the

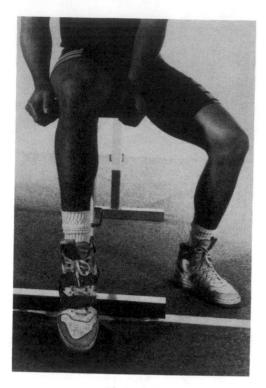

Photo 1.3

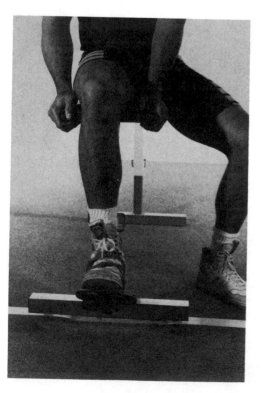

Photo 1.4

bar of a barbell across your toes. Hold the barbell in place and raise your toes (the front of the foot) as high as possible. Keep holding the bar in place and lower your toes as far as possible and then raise as high as possible.

Variant 2: This exercise is done with an iron boot or foot harness secured to the bottom of the foot. With the resistance in place, sit on the edge of a high bench so that your leg hangs straight down from the knees (see Photo 1.3). Lower the toe-ball area of your foot as much as possible. When you are ready, raise the front of your foot as high as possible (see Photo 1.4). Relax the muscles, return to the down position, and repeat.

Comments

- It is important to understand that you cannot raise your foot much above the horizontal position. Thus, it is important that you go through the maximum range of motion below the horizontal.
- Specialized exercise machines are available for doing dorsi flexion, but they are usually found in the offices of physical therapists or athletic trainers. However, the two variants described are very effective. Keep in mind that the dorsi flexors are much weaker than the plantar flexors and great weights are not needed. Thus, a relatively small amount of weight will give you a very strong workout.

■ Seated Calf Raise (Seated Heel Raise)

Many people do the seated calf raise (seated heel raise) in the belief that it develops both the gastrocnemius and soleus muscles. However, this is not so. The gastrocnemius is not strongly involved in the seated calf raise.

Major muscles and actions involved

The soleus is the only major muscle involved in performing ankle joint extension (plantar flexion) in the seated calf raise (see Figure 1.6). In this exercise, ankle joint extension raises the heels while the balls of the feet remain in contact with the foot platform.

Sports uses

The seated calf raise and the muscles involved are very important in all running and jumping

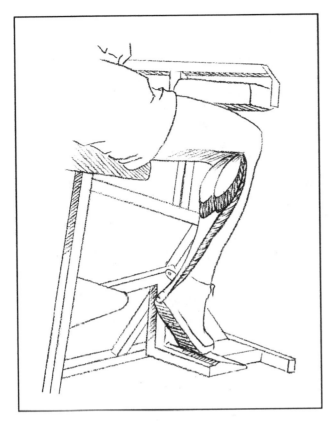

Figure 1.6
Muscles used in the seated calf raise

type activities. See the section on the heel raise for more information.

In addition, it should be emphasized that the seated calf raise is very important for all long-distance or endurance-type activities. The soleus has great staying power and the more you can develop it, the longer it will enable you to continue an activity. The gastrocnemius is usually composed of mainly white fibers or an equal amount of white and red fibers. Thus, the soleus can take over in many cases when the gastrocnemius becomes fatigued. For this reason it is very important that the soleus be developed together with the gastrocnemius. It should also be pointed out that the soleus is most important in giving width to the calf muscles.

Execution

It is most effective and convenient to perform seated calf raises on specialized exercise machines such as the one made by Keiser. To prepare for this exercise, assume a seated position and place your feet on the angled foot

platform. Make sure the balls of your feet are in full contact with the platform and that your heels are free to move.

When you are seated, grasp the handles (on which you adjust the resistance) and pull the padded stabilizing bar over your lower thighs. When positioned, adjust the resistance. Then inhale slightly more than usual and hold your breath as you raise your heels as high as possible (see Photos 1.5 and 1.6). Exhale and relax slightly and lower your heels under control to the initial position below the level of the balls of the feet. Repeat at the desired tempo.

Comments

- The soleus muscle has great muscular endurance. This is seen when the action is repeated for a period of time or when the contraction is held for several or more seconds. Because of this, for greater development you should do some holding in the top position or any intermediate position. With the Keiser machine you can increase (or decrease) the resistance at any point in the range of motion during the up or down phase. This allows you to develop strength at any point or over the full range of motion.
- The seated calf raise is an excellent exercise for development of the soleus muscle. And, because it is a very strong muscle, you can use great resistance. Keep in mind that the soleus together with the gastrocnemius can exert over 1,000 pounds of force. However, that does not mean that you can raise this amount, because other factors are involved. Thus, you should not start with extremely heavy weights: Start slowly and gradually increase the amount of resistance that you use. Keep in mind that a maximum range of motion is very important for full development of the muscle-tendon arrangement.
- To develop some of the assisting muscles and to bring in some other foot actions, you should change foot positions. For example, point your toes inward and then rise up. This positioning will force some inversion and produce more development of the tibialis posterior (along with the muscles used in ankle joint extension). Pointing your toes outward and then doing toe raises will use foot eversion and the muscles involved (the peroneal and the extensor digitorum longus muscles located on the lateral sides of the lower legs). Placing your feet

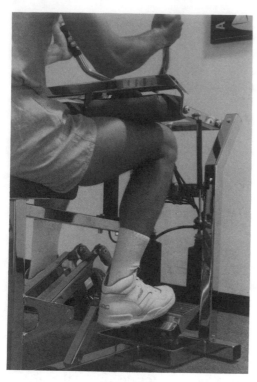

Photo 1.5

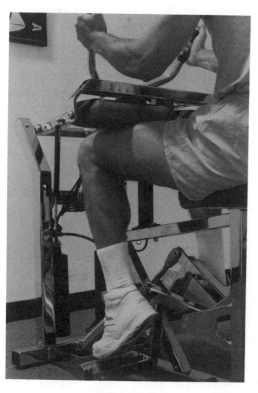

Photo 1.6

slightly wider apart or closer together will also produce greater all-around development.

• To get a greater stretch of the Achilles tendon and soleus muscle, it is important that the foot placement platform be angled downward as on the Keiser machine. This initial prior stretching is very important for a stronger return contraction. It also allows for a greater range of motion, which is so important in running and jumping.

• When using the Keiser calf machine, the exercise can be performed at a wide variety of speeds, from very slow to fast. This feature is not available on other machines, which limits their value to some extent, mainly for athletes. By doing the exercise very fast, you are able to develop some of the white fibers, which are usually not predominant in the soleus muscle, which is mainly a red muscle used for endurance-type activities. However, doing the exercise at both slow and fast speeds is very effective and produces slightly different results.

• If a seated calf raise machine is not available, the exercise can be done with a weighted barbell. In this case, assume a seated position on an exercise bench and place the balls of your feet on a wooden block approximately 2–4 inches high. Be sure the block is sufficiently stable to prevent it from tipping and causing an injury. When you are in position, place the barbell across your lower thighs. Raise your heels up and down as described.

2 The Knee Joint

ANATOMY OF THE KNEE

The knee is a very unstable and complex joint. It is formed by the articulation of the femur (thigh bone) with the fibula and tibia bones of the shin. The knee joint is a hinge joint and its action is similar to the movement of a door on hinges. However, it is not a true hinge joint because some rotation and sliding of the bones is possible when the knee is bent.

The knee joint is stabilized and held together by many ligaments and tendons. The ligaments also play an important role in limiting the range of motion in the joint. If they did not perform this function, the bones of the knee joint would literally pop apart when you assume the extreme position of flexion as in a deep squat.

Your knees must not only support your weight, but must also be used so that you can walk, run, jump, and so on. In addition, the knees play a major role in shock absorbing during jumping and running. Because of this and because the knee is anatomically unstable, it is very important that you develop all of the muscles around the knee.

BASIC MOVEMENTS OF THE KNEE

The basic movements of the knee joint are flexion and extension. In flexion the shin moves back and up, that is, the back of the shin moves toward the back of the thigh, or the back of the thigh moves toward the shin. An example of the latter is the movement of going down in the squat.

In extension (the opposite of flexion) the shin moves away from the thigh or vice versa and the leg is straightened. When the knee is fully extended, the knee joint is locked in place and no rotation is possible. However, when the knee is flexed, the lower leg can be rotated in or out, but the range of movement is small. Rotation is used most often in the movement of pushing off and turning the body in a different direction.

MAJOR MUSCLES INVOLVED

There are 12 muscles which act on the knee joint. They can be classified in three distinct groups: 1) the quadriceps femoris group, located on the anterior (front) side of the thigh (see Figure 2.1); 2) the hamstring muscle group, located on the posterior (back) side of the thigh (see Figure 2.2); and 3) a combination of muscles that assist mostly in flexion and inward rotation. The quadriceps muscle group includes the rectus femoris, vastus lateralis, vastus medialis, and vastus intermedius muscles, which extend the knee.

The vastus muscles run almost the entire length of the femur and converge into the quadriceps femoris tendon, which attaches to the patella bone (kneecap). The vastus lateralis is a large muscle located halfway down the outer side of the thigh. It originates on the lateral surface of the femur from just below the upper head of the bone to almost the lower end.

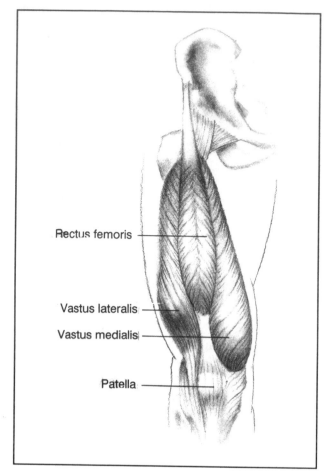

Figure 2.1
Anterior view of the upper right leg (thigh)

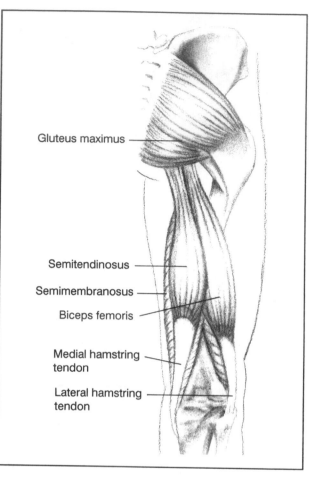

Figure 2.2
Posterior view of the upper right leg (thigh)

The vastus medialis is located on the medial (inner) side of the thigh, somewhat lower than the lateralis, and is partially covered by the rectus femoris. It originates on the medial side of almost the entire shaft of the femur.

The vastus intermedius is a close associate of the vastus medialis and lateralis. It lies between them and beneath the rectus femoris. It is difficult to see this muscle separate from the medialis and often the two are continuous for part of their length. The vastus intermedius originates on the anterior and lateral sides of the femur, running almost the entire length of the shaft of the femur.

The rectus femoris is a large muscle positioned straight down the front of the thigh. It originates on the spine of the ilium bone of the pelvic girdle. Because of this attachment, it has an action at the hip joint as well as the knee joint.

At the lower end the rectus femoris joins the tendons of the four vastus muscles merging together onto the patella bone and surrounding ligaments. The patella, however, is a free-floating bone and attaches to the tibia via the patella ligament. This ligament, for all practical purposes, acts as though it were a tendon.

The hamstring muscle group includes the semitendinosus, the semimembranosus, and the biceps femoris. These muscles flex the knee. The biceps femoris is the largest muscle of the hamstring group and has two heads. At the upper end the long head is attached to the tuberosity of the ischium bone of the pelvic girdle. The short head is attached to the middle and central area of the femur bone of the thigh. At the lower end the biceps femoris is attached to the lateral condyle of the tibia and the head of the fibula bones of the shin. The tendon of insertion (which attaches to the bone) forms the lateral hamstring.

The semitendinosus runs from the tuberosity of the ischium (on a common tendon with the biceps femoris) to the upper medial condyle of the tibia. The semimembranosus also attaches to the tuberosity of the ischium at the upper end and to the posterior medial condyle of the tibia at the lower end. Both the semimembranosus and semitendinosus extend the thigh and assist in hip joint medial rotation. Because their tendon of insertion is on the medial side of the knee joint, they are known as the medial hamstrings.

The semimembranosus and semitendinosus muscles lie side by side on the inside back of the thigh. They are much thinner than the biceps femoris and have a unique relationship. The semimembranosus has a long upper tendon and a short lower tendon, and the semitendinosus has a short upper tendon and a long lower tendon. Because of this, the muscle masses of each of these muscles are in line with one another and form a cylindrical mass. Therefore, when well developed they appear as one long muscle.

The hamstring muscle is a two-joint muscle having an action at the knee and hip joints. These actions can be separated—in other words, the knee can act independently of the hip joint and the muscles can act to produce movement in only one of the joints. It is interesting to note that when both ends of the muscle act simultaneously, the contraction of the muscle is weaker than when only one end is involved.

Other muscles which also act on the knee are the sartorius, the gracilis, the popliteus, the gastrocnemius, and the plantaris. However, because they are not major muscles in their action at the knee, they will not be discussed here.

KNEE JOINT EXERCISES

■ Knee Extension (Leg Extension)

Most bodybuilders and athletes use the squat exercise as the main exercise for the anterior thighs (the quadriceps femoris muscle group). Although the squat is an excellent exercise, it does have shortcomings. For example, the main developmental phase of the squat is the early rise out of the down position. When the legs are almost straight, the quadriceps is still involved but not strongly. Because of this, you never get full development of the vastus medialis, which is very important in the prevention of chondromalacia.

To target this important muscle but still involve the knee extensors, you should do knee extensions (leg extensions). The most effective machine for execution is the one made by Keiser, which allows you to do the exercise at different speeds and with varying intensities on both the concentric and eccentric contractions. However, the basic execution is the same on all machines.

Major muscles and actions involved

In the knee joint there is extension, which involves the quadriceps femoris muscle group (see Figure 2.3). In this action the shin moves away from the thigh until the leg is completely straightened (locked).

Sports uses

Knee extension and the muscles involved are needed for the execution of many basic skills including jumping, running, kicking, skipping, lifting, and pushing. More specifically, knee joint extension is needed in all of the jump events such as the high jump, long jump, and pole vault; in the jump shot and rebounding in basketball; and in the spike and block in volleyball. In running, knee joint extensor muscles prevent "sitting," stabilize the knee, and participate in the push-off.

Knee extensions are important in football, baseball, softball, soccer, rugby, basketball, lacrosse, tennis, racquetball, and many other sports. Knee joint extension is also very important in kicking in sports such as football, soccer, and karate and other martial arts. It also plays a major role in the lunging and cutting actions used in almost all movement sports.

Knee joint extension is one of the main actions in lifting weights off the floor, as, for example, in the deadlift and squat events in the sport of powerlifting, and in the snatch and clean and jerk events in weightlifting. For bodybuilders, knee joint extension is one of the major exercises used for developing and defining the anterior thigh muscles.

Execution

Assume a seated position on the leg extension machine so that your knees are at the end of the

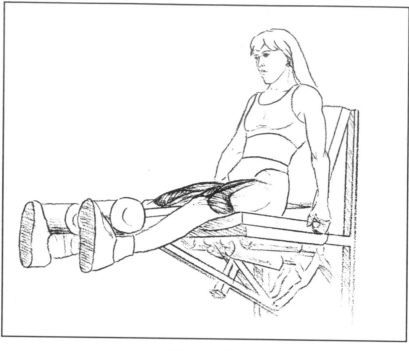

Figure 2.3
Muscles used in knee extension (leg extension)

bench and your lower legs hang vertically at a 90-degree angle. Adjust the seat height and back support so that you can place the insteps and base of your shins against the inner side of the resistance arm rollers. Sit upright (more difficult) or lean your trunk back to approximately a 45-degree angle and hold onto the grips alongside the bench with your hands (see Photo 2.1).

When you are in position on the Keiser machine, adjust the resistance. On most standard machines this must be done before you sit down. When you are ready, take a slightly greater than normal breath and then hold your breath as you push against the bottom roller with your lower legs. Push the rollers forward and up until your knee joints are completely extended and locked. Your legs should be straight and rigid (see Photo 2.2). Relax the muscles somewhat and exhale as you return to the initial position under control. Stop when there is a 90-degree angle in your knee joint and then repeat.

Comments

• When using the Keiser leg extension machine, you have several additional options. You can work your legs unilaterally or alternately. In this way, if one of your legs is weaker than the other, you can do additional work with the weaker leg until your legs are balanced. Even more important, when using the Keiser machine you can change the resistance (air pressure) during execution, which allows you to adjust the resistance to your needs. For example, you can increase the resistance at your sticking point to do an isometric contraction and then reduce the pressure to continue the movement to lock out. In addition, you can increase the resistance on the return to create a greater eccentric load.

• Athletes, and at times bodybuilders, use the Keiser machine to do high-speed movements which are not possible on other machines. These leg extension machines maintain a smooth, consistent resistance curve over a wide range of speeds. High-speed movements are very effective for hitting the more explosive white fibers, which are most important in almost all sports. However, other machines can only be used at slow or moderate speeds.

It should also be pointed out that when using the Keiser machine unilaterally, you can alternate the leg movements at a fast speed to simulate various sports. When alternating, each leg has a short period of time in which to slightly recuperate before the next maximal contraction. However, performing the exercise very fast should be done only for short periods of time, up to about 10–15 seconds. After this time your ATP stores are more or less depleted and you should rest until they are replenished before repeating.

- For most bodybuilders and especially athletes, it is important that the angle in the knee joint be 90 degrees (measured from the back of the thigh to the back of the shin) when doing the exercise. If the angle is less than 90 degrees, that is, when the shin is under the thigh, a great amount of stress is placed on the knee joint at the start of the extension movement. If light weights are used there is no problem. However, when heavy weights are used the tension can cause severe injury to the knee in this extreme knee-flexed position. Because of this, you should work in this range only if you are physically prepared.

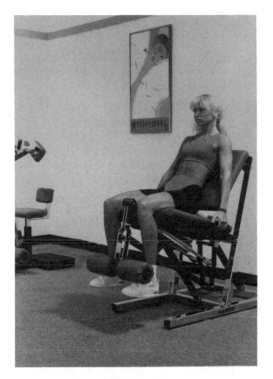

Photo 2.1

- The backward lean of the trunk is needed to get more involvement of the rectus femoris muscle. When you are seated in an upright position, your hip is flexed, which produces slack in the upper end of this muscle. By leaning back you put the muscle more on stretch, which, when it contracts at the lower end, will create more tension. Trunk positioning, whether it be upright or a backward lean, does not play a role in the development of the vastus muscles. These muscles do not cross the hip joint and, therefore, are effectively involved regardless of trunk position.

- The knee extension exercise is excellent for isolation of the quadriceps femoris muscle group. In this exercise no other muscles are involved in extending the lower leg. Because of this, knee extensions, especially on the Keiser machine, are used a great deal in rehabilitation or for athletes who do not have adequate strength for proper execution of more difficult exercises. They allow the muscles involved to be exercised with controlled loading without any of the difficulties typically found when doing squats or lunges. Also, it is the only exercise that allows for safe locking-out of the knee joint. In squats, lunges, and leg presses, the compression forces are too great.

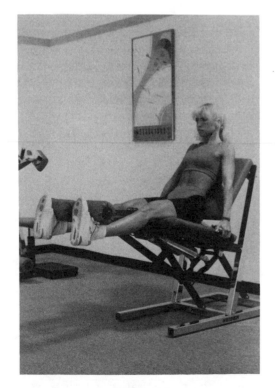

Photo 2.2

■ Knee Curl

Most sports actions and normal everyday activities such as walking and running rely mostly on the anterior thigh muscles. However, in order to have a truly strong knee, which is involved in so many activities, it is also necessary to balance the development of the quadriceps muscles with development of the hamstrings on the posterior side. One of the best exercises for the lower portion of the hamstrings is the knee curl when done on a machine such as the one by Keiser.

Major muscles and actions involved

Knee curls involve mainly the lower portion of the hamstring muscle group on the back side of the thighs (see Figure 2.4). The action in this exercise is knee joint flexion, in which the back of the shin moves toward the back of the thigh.

It must be understood that the hamstring muscle, because it crosses both joints, does not contract maximally at both ends when an exercise is being done at the knee or hip. Thus, the knee curl exercise involves the lower hamstring. That does not mean that the hamstring is divided into different parts. It is not. The hamstring muscle is one long, continuous muscle. But the activity is greatest at the lower end in this exercise.

Sports uses

Active knee joint flexion is used in running and kicking to "fold" the shin under the thigh as the leg is brought forward in the main action phase. It is needed in back kicks in soccer and in various wrestling moves. Aerialists use this action a great deal when hanging from their knees on the trapeze, and dancers need it to bring their shins up in various jumps. For bodybuilders, the knee curl is a key exercise for the development of the middle and lower back of the thigh. Doing knee curls is also very important in preventing knee injuries.

Execution

The knee curl exercise can be done lying face down or in a standing position. Because of the greater availability and ease of execution, the lying knee curl exercise on the Keiser machine will be described. Execution is basically the same on other machines.

Assume a face-down position on a lying knee curl machine so that your knees extend over the end of the bench and are free of support. The back of your lower leg (upper ankle) should rest against the underside of the rollers. Hold the grips alongside the bench to hold your upper body in place and to adjust the resistance (see Photo 2.3).

When you are ready, take a slightly greater than normal breath and then hold your breath as you raise your feet by bending your knee. In the ending position, your shins should be slightly past the vertical position (see Photo 2.4). Exhale and relax the muscles as you return to the original position under control and repeat. Execute at a moderate rate of speed. However, when using the Keiser machine, you can also do the exercise quickly. In addition, you can do the exercise with one leg only or in an alternating fashion for variety.

In the standing knee curl exercise you can use a specialized machine or a weight boot (shoe). Execution is basically the same as in the lying down variant. However, when using a weighted

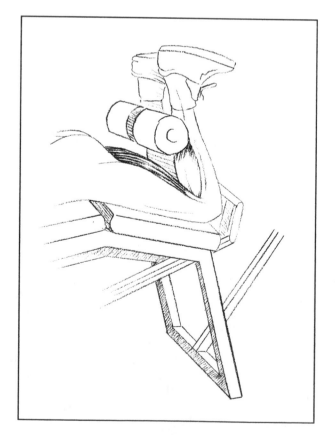

Figure 2.4
Muscles used in the knee curl

boot you will also involve slight hip joint flexion to assist the knee joint action.

Comments

- The knee curl exercise is very important for stabilizing the knee and preventing injury. In addition, hamstring development is important to balance the quadriceps, which should always be stronger. However, the exact ratio of strength between the quadriceps and hamstrings has not been determined with any degree of accuracy. It seems reasonable to expect greater strength of the quadriceps, however, since this muscle group is substantially larger and is used in more activities. Thus a 3:1 or even a 4:1 ratio is usually recommended. It is also interesting to note that some studies have shown that the stronger the hamstrings are, the more the quadriceps can be developed. Therefore, always complement quadriceps work with hamstring exercises.

- In the lying knee curl exercise, when heavy weights are used the pelvic girdle has a tendency to rise up (hip joint flexion). This happens naturally to raise the upper attachment of the hamstring muscles so that they are more taut and thus become more effective as knee joint flexors.

  Excessive raising of the pelvic girdle is potentially harmful to the lower back because the lumbar spine undergoes hyperextension during the movement. Because the movement is passive, it creates excessive pinching (pressure) on the posterior spinal discs. If the pressure is great enough, in time it can cause injury.

  To alleviate this situation, you should use an angled bench such as depicted on the Keiser machine. When you lie down, the bench automatically places the hip joint in flexion. Such positioning not only takes the pressure off the lumbar vertebrae and discs, but it also raises the attachment of the upper hamstrings to provide for a more effective pull of the muscles.

- The knee curl exercise is most effective for development of the lower hamstrings, especially the short head of the biceps femoris muscle, which does not cross the hip joint. It is not effective for development of the upper end of the hamstrings. The reason for this is twofold. First, as exercise intensity increases, hip joint flexion occurs and the upper hamstring must stretch, not shorten, in its contrac-

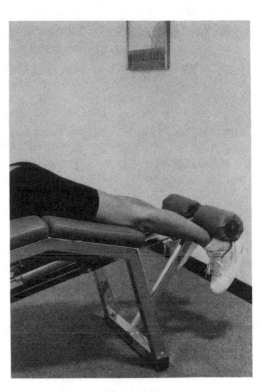

Photo 2.3

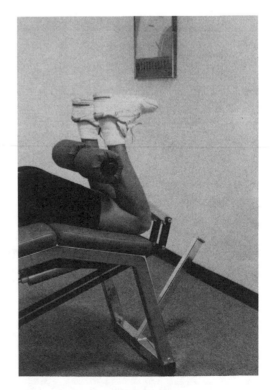

Photo 2.4

tion. Second, because the upper end is responsible for hip joint extension, it must be exercised in this action. Therefore, you must do hip joint extensions to develop the upper fibers.

- To develop both the upper and lower ends of the hamstrings maximally in one exercise, glute-ham-gastroc raises should be performed. (This exercise is described in Chapter 4.)

3 The Hip Joint and Pelvic Girdle

ANATOMY OF THE HIP JOINT AND PELVIC GIRDLE

Each half (side) of the pelvic girdle consists of three bones: the ilium, which is located at the top and sides of the hip; the pubis, which is below and in front; and the ischium, which is below and to the rear.

The pelvic basin is closed on the back side by the sacrum (the lower end of the spine), which is wedged between the two ilium (hip) bones and held together by the strongest ligaments in the body. This is commonly known as the sacroiliac joint, which is often involved in back pain.

The hip joint is formed by the head of the femur (thigh bone) articulating in the acetabulum, a deep socket formed on the outer surface of the pelvis where the ilium, pubis, and ischium bones join together. The hip joint is a ball-and-socket joint, which means that the leg can rotate in all directions inside the socket. Strong ligaments surround and hold the joint together and limit the amount of movement that is possible in the joint, usually to 30–45 degrees from the anatomical position (when the legs and body form a straight line).

In this arrangement the thigh can move in only a limited range of motion when the pelvic girdle is held stationary. When the pelvis also rotates, the leg can be raised through a greater range of motion. In most movements of the leg there is a combination of both thigh and pelvic movement.

When the leg is stationary, movement of the pelvis increases the range of motion of the trunk in all directions. Thus, the pelvis plays an important role in many movements.

BASIC MOVEMENTS OF THE HIP JOINT

Six major movements occur in the hip joint. They are: 1) flexion, 2) extension, 3) adduction, 4) abduction, 5) medial rotation, and 6) lateral rotation. Because the hip is a ball-and-socket joint, circumduction can also occur. However, this latter movement is rarely, if ever, used in sports and will not be discussed.

1. Hip joint flexion: Movement of the thigh forward is called flexion. When you are in a standing position, flexion occurs when the leg is raised forward and upward approximately 150 degrees or more. When the leg is bent, the mass of the trunk will stop hip joint flexion. However, when the leg is kept straight, the tightness of the hamstrings will determine how much flexion can be exhibited in the hip joint.

2. Hip joint extension: Extension is the reverse of flexion. In this action the leg is brought down and back to the anatomical straight-line body position from a hip-flexed position. When the leg reaches a vertical position, it is stopped in its movement by the tension of the ligaments and the psoas and iliacus muscles. Because of this, hyperextension in the hip

19

joint is not possible except in rare, abnormal cases. Hyperextension can occur, however, when the leg is brought behind the body because when this is done, the anterior pelvis tilts forward.

3. Hip joint adduction: In hip joint adduction one leg is moved toward the other leg (toward the midline of the body) from an out-to-the-sides position. Adduction is limited when the moving leg makes contact with the support leg. When the leg is brought across the midline of the body, the pelvis on the side of the non-support leg must be rotated and dropped so that, in essence, adduction in the hip joint opposite the moving leg occurs.

4. Hip joint abduction: In hip joint abduction, the leg is moved from the midline out toward the side of the body. The usual range of motion is approximately 45 degrees or more—the exact amount depends upon the tightness of the opposing muscles.

5. Medial rotation: In medial (inward) hip joint rotation, the femur is rotated inward. The amount of rotation is limited when the neck of the femur hits the rim of the acetabulum.

6. Lateral rotation: In lateral (outward) rotation, the leg is rotated outward. In this movement the femur rotates away from the other leg.

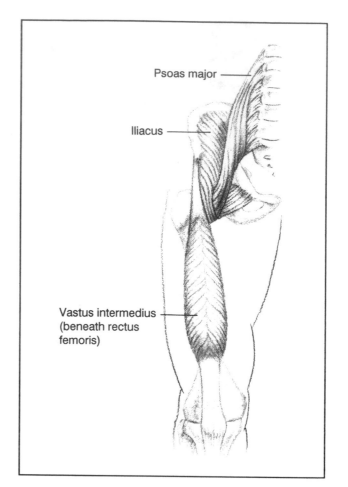

Figure 3.1
Anterior view of the right leg (thigh and hip)

MAJOR MUSCLES INVOLVED

Hip joint flexion

The major muscles involved in hip joint flexion are the psoas, the iliacus, the pectineus, and the rectus femoris (see Figure 3.1). The psoas lies in the abdominal cavity behind the internal organs and cannot be seen. It originates on the sides of the last thoracic and all the lumbar vertebrae. At the lower end the psoas attaches to the lesser trochanter of the femur.

It is important to understand that the psoas attaches to the lumbar vertebrae. Because of this, when you are lying down and you raise your legs, the psoas not only pulls on the femur to lift the legs, but it also pulls on the lower vertebrae. When this occurs spinal hyperextension can result if the abdominal muscles are not strongly contracted to counteract this effect.

The iliacus is a flat, triangular muscle that originates on the inner surface of the ilium and part of the inner surface of the sacrum near the ilium. Its tendon of insertion joins that of the psoas just in front of the pelvis and attaches on the femur. Because of the common tendon, the psoas and iliacus are known as the iliopsoas.

The rectus femoris is a large muscle that runs straight down the front of the thigh, as discussed in Chapter 2.

Hip joint extension

The major muscles involved in hip joint extension are the hamstring muscle group and the gluteus maximus. The hamstring is composed of three muscles: the biceps femoris, the semitendinosus, and the semimembranosus.

The gluteus maximus is a very large, fleshy muscle at the back of the hip (the one you sit on).

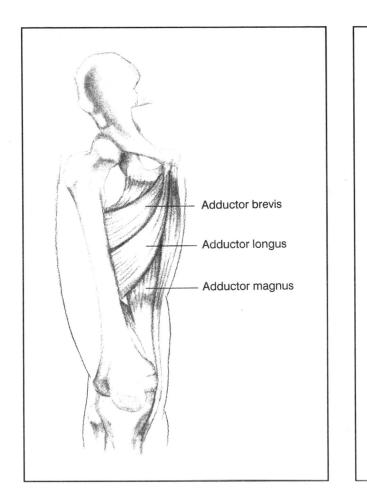

Figure 3.2
The right thigh: adductor muscles

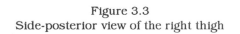

Figure 3.3
Side-posterior view of the right thigh

It originates on the outer surface of the crest of the ilium, the posterior surface of the sacrum near the ilium, the fascia of the lumbar area, and the sides of the coccyx. It inserts on a broad line about four inches high on the posterior side of the femur and the iliotibial tract of the fascia latae.

The gluteus maximus is involved mainly in extension and outward rotation. The upper fibers also assist in abduction, and the lower fibers assist in adduction.

Hip joint adduction

The adductor longus, brevis, and magnus, and the gracilis are involved in hip joint adduction (see Figure 3.2).

The adductor magnus, situated on the medial (inner) side of the thigh, is one of the largest muscles of the body. It originates on the front of the pubis, the tuberosity of the ischium, and the length of the ramus connecting them. Insertion is on the whole length of the linea aspera of the femur. The adductor brevis is a short, triangular muscle behind and above the adductor longus. It originates on the ramus of the pubis and inserts on the upper half of the linea aspera of the femur. The adductor longus lies just to the inner side of the pectineus. It begins on the front of the pubis and ends on the linea aspera in the middle third of the femur.

The gracilis is a long, slender muscle which passes down the inner side of the thigh. It originates on the lower half of the symphysis pubis and the upper half of the pubic arch. It inserts on the upper part of the medial surface of the tibia (below the knee). It also assists with flexion and inward rotation.

Hip joint abduction

The gluteus medius is the major muscle involved in hip joint abduction (see Figure 3.3). It is a short, thick muscle located at the sides of the ilium and gives the rounded contour to the sides of the hip. It originates on the outer surface of the ilium near its crest and inserts on the lateral surface of the greater trochanter of the femur. The anterior fibers assist with inward rotation and flexion and the posterior fibers assist with outward rotation and extension.

HIP JOINT EXERCISES

Hip exercises are usually performed by women, who use them in an effort to shape the hips, but these exercises are also extremely important for all athletes and bodybuilders.

The most effective way of doing hip exercises has always been with a pulley type system. Today, however, with the advent of hip exercise machines, execution is safer and, in some cases, more effective.

■ Hip Joint Flexion

Hip flexion exercises are extremely important for athletes because the muscles they develop play a very important role in spinal stability. When the hip flexor muscles and the hip extensor muscles are both strong and flexible, the pelvis will be properly positioned to balance the spine effectively.

Major muscles and actions involved

The iliopsoas, pectineus, and rectus femoris muscles are involved in hip flexion (see Figure 3.4). In this exercise the thigh is brought forward and up from a position behind the body.

Sports uses

The action of hip flexion and the muscles involved are very important in all sports that require sprinting, kicking, and quick stepping out to get to a ball or opponent. In sprinting or running this action is needed to bring the swing leg forward quickly for greater stride length and to prepare for stronger backward movement. In sports such as basketball, volleyball, baseball,

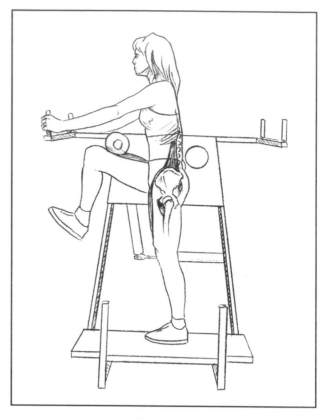

Figure 3.4
Muscles used in hip joint flexion

football, rugby, hockey, and soccer, hip flexion is very important in running and for that quick first step when reaching (stepping) forward. Hip flexion plays an important role in bringing the thigh forward to produce greater force in soccer and football kicking.

Execution

Hip joint flexion is most easily and effectively executed on a multi-hip machine such as the one made by Keiser. To position yourself properly, stand on the foot platform with your side facing the machine. Adjust the height of the foot platform so that your hip joint is in line with the axis of the resistance lever arm. Set the resistance pad so that it is at five o'clock if you face the seven o'clock position (when exercising the right leg). When you are properly positioned, hold the grip handles (which also control the air resistance) and adjust the pressure. When you are ready, your body should be erect and the leg to be exercised should be bent and slightly behind your body (see Photo 3.1).

At this time, inhale slightly more than usual and hold your breath as you pull your thigh forward up to the horizontal or slightly above the horizontal position (see Photo 3.2). Keep your knee bent to allow for maximum range of motion. After reaching the uppermost position, exhale as you return to the starting position.

Keep your trunk erect and your support leg straight during the entire execution. Pause momentarily in the bottom position and then repeat. When you finish exercising one leg, turn around, reset the resistance lever arm, and repeat with the opposite leg.

Comments

- To allow for effective stretching and full-range development of the muscles, it is critical that you maintain an erect upper-body position. When you do this while your leg is brought to the rear, you should feel a stretch of the hip flexors on the leg being exercised. This pre-stretching utilizes the stretch reflex, which produces a stronger contraction in the power phase. If you incline your trunk forward as your leg returns to the rear, you will not get the stretch in the muscles and you will be using the inertia of the upper body to bring the thigh forward. This defeats the value of the exercise.
- Raising your thigh as high as possible is not necessary in this exercise unless you are looking for additional abdominal development. It is important to understand that the hip flexors are strongly involved in the initial pull in this exercise. However, because of the ligamentous structure of the hip, the thigh can be raised only approximately 45-60 degrees past the vertical. When you raise the thigh higher, the pelvic girdle must rotate backwards. To do this, the abdominals, especially the lower abdominals, must undergo concentric contraction.
- The Keiser machine allows you to bring your thigh through very quickly from the behind-the-back position. This action closely duplicates the action used in running and jumping, thereby allowing you to do a sport-specific exercise to improve your performance. Also, after you bring your thigh forward, you can straighten your leg as done in high jumping, or you can keep it bent to achieve maximum height. Even more importantly, you can immediately reverse direction in the bottom position to do fast multiple repetitions. This helps to

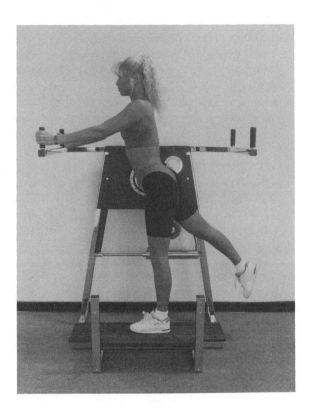

Photo 3.1

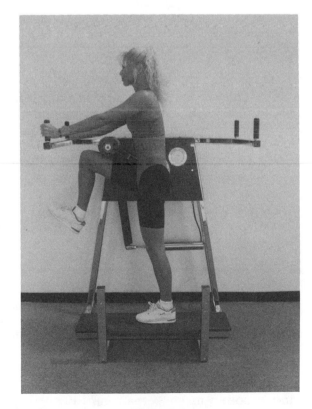

Photo 3.2

develop the explosive contraction of the hip flexor muscles. In addition, the Keiser machine lets you regulate the amount of resistance throughout the entire range of motion. Thus you can do isometric contractions in mid-range or at any other point or create a strong eccentric return to develop the muscles in this manner.

- Hip flexion can also be executed on a low pulley machine. In this variant you must have an assistant for support to maintain the erect position. To execute, place a cuff around your ankle, face away from the pulley, and pull your thigh through in the same manner as on the multi-hip machine. Be careful not to kick the person you are leaning on for support.

■ Hip Joint Extension

To develop the gluteus maximus and the upper portion of the hamstring muscles, most bodybuilders and athletes do squats and lunges. However, most of the visible results of these exercises are in the quadriceps because most people do not squat or lunge deeply enough to maximally tax the gluteus maximus. To remedy this situation, you should do straight-leg hip extensions, an excellent exercise for the gluteus maximus.

Major muscles and actions involved

The gluteus maximus and the upper hamstring muscles are involved in hip joint extension (see Figure 3.5). It must be understood that the hamstrings are continuous muscles. However, in this exercise only the upper portion undergoes great electrical activity and shortening. The lower end is relatively quiet. In hip joint extension the leg moves backward from a forward (hip-flexed) position until it is slightly behind the body.

Sports uses

Hip joint extension and the muscles involved are very important in the execution of many basic skills such as jumping for height or distance; all forms of running, skipping, leaping, and lifting; and pushing with the lower body.

More specifically, hip joint extension is needed in sports such as track and field, rebounding and shooting in basketball, and blocking and spiking in volleyball. In running, hip joint exten-

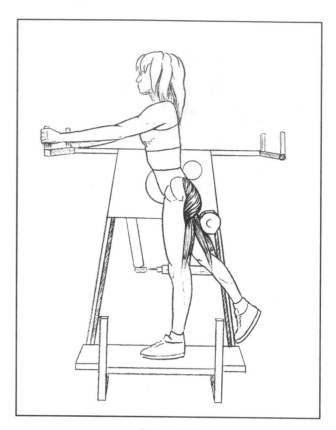

Figure 3.5
Muscles used in hip joint extension

sion is the main action in the "paw-back," which pushes the runner forward after a touchdown. Running and jumping are needed in the sports of track, football, baseball, soccer, rugby, team handball, basketball, tennis, lacrosse, and many other sports.

Hip joint extension is also very important in lifting weights off the floor, especially in the deadlift and squat events in powerlifting and in the clean portion of the weightlifting events. Bodybuilders need this exercise to develop and define the buttocks muscles.

Execution

Execution of hip joint extension is most effective on a multi-hip machine such as the one made by Keiser. To use such machines properly, the height of the foot platform must be adjusted so that your hip joint lines up with the axis of the resistance lever arm as your side faces the machine. Then adjust the resistance roller to the eight or nine o'clock hour when exercising the right leg. Place the leg to be exercised on top of the roller so that it is in a maximally hip-flexed position. Hold onto the handles, which also control the resistance on the Keiser machine.

When you are in a stable position with your support leg straight and your upper body erect, you are ready to begin the exercise (see Photo 3.3). Inhale slightly more than usual and hold your breath as you push down on the lever arm until your leg is slightly behind your body (see Photo 3.4). Keep your trunk erect at all times. Exhale and relax your muscles slightly as you return to the initial position and then repeat.

Comments

- On the standard multi-hip machines you must stop in the up position before beginning the return. This is effective for developing muscle strength. However, the Keiser machine allows you to do quick reversals, which help to develop the resiliency of the hip joint extensors that is most important in the running and jumping sports. To execute the exercise in this manner, after returning to the hip-flexed starting position, quickly reverse the movement of your leg and pull all the way down and back as quickly as possible. The return to the starting position can be done relatively slowly, but the reversal and the down action should be done very quickly. Other machines do not allow you to do quick reversals and fast movements.

- To more closely duplicate the paw-back action in running, which is one of the key actions in propelling the body forward, you should straighten your leg as you begin the downward movement. On the return to the initial position, bend your knee and then straighten it as you go downward in a continuous manner. This is also a critical action that hurdlers use when getting back into the running pattern after clearing the hurdle.

- Maintaining an erect body position is very important for proper execution. If you lean forward as your leg is being pulled down and back, you will be using body momentum and an isometric contraction of the muscles being exercised. When you maintain the erect position, the muscle will be used through the full range of motion.

- It should also be noted that when your leg passes the vertical position, that is, when it is directly under your body, your pelvic girdle must rotate anteriorly to allow the leg to go to

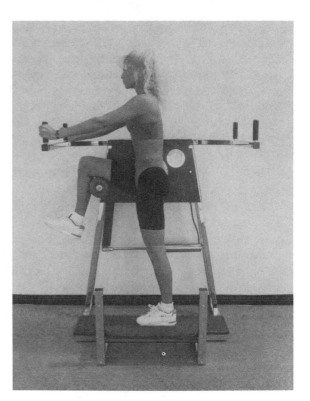

Photo 3.3

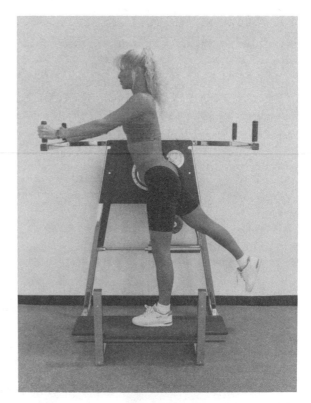

Photo 3.4

the rear. This is an important feature in many sports, such as running, that allows you to create an effective and long-duration push-off. However, note that the muscles involved in rotating the pelvis are the erector spinae muscles of the lower back. The hip extensor muscles remain under isometric contraction to keep the leg and pelvic girdle working as one unit.

• The Keiser machine allows you to increase or decrease the resistance at any point in the range of motion. Thus you can increase the resistance in the initial range of motion or in mid-range to more closely duplicate the actions used in your particular sport. In addition, you can increase the resistance on the return to create a stronger eccentric contraction, especially as your leg achieves a more flexed position. This is very important for greater resiliency and for generating more power on the initial hip-joint extension. This is most important for weightlifters and for running and jumping actions in other sports.

• In essence, the Keiser hip extension machine can be used to duplicate all the different types of muscular contractions needed in your particular sport. In this regard note that if you injure yourself, the resistance can be adjusted to match your capabilities while you are rehabilitating your hamstring muscles.

• Hip extension can also be done on a high pulley system. In this case you must start with your leg extended and horizontal, that is, perpendicular to the vertical support leg. You then pull down with your leg held straight to a position directly below the body or slightly to the rear. Athletes can usually do this exercise without support, but if the exercise is new to you, you should have someone alongside you for support. Note that only single repetitions can be done with a high pulley.

When using a pulley or a hip extension machine, it is important that you do not pull your leg as far to the rear as possible. When you do this you are severely rotating your pelvic girdle forward, which creates excessive hyperextension in your lower spine. This can accentuate swayback and create lower back problems. More important, it must be understood that the gluteus maximus is most effectively worked when you start with your leg in a flexed position.

• Although this exercise involves the erector spinae muscle group, these muscles are used in only a secondary action. Because of this, you should not lock your hips to force the erectors to do the work.

■ Hip Joint Adduction

The hip adductor muscles are some of the largest in the body. In a way this is surprising because few actions used in normal activities or even in sports activities truly require hip adduction, especially when it is executed with a great deal of force. Most likely, these muscles are strong to create a stable internal base for the pelvis and, even more important, to aid in rotational movements of the body when the leg is held in place on the floor. Thus it is important to develop these muscles, and one of the best exercises for this is hip adduction.

Major muscles and movements involved

In hip joint adduction one or both legs are pulled in toward the midline of the body from an abducted (out to the side) position. These actions involve the adductor longus, brevis, and magnus and the gracilis muscles (see Figure 3.6).

Sports uses

Hip joint adduction is very useful in sports which require court maneuvering such as tennis, racquetball, basketball, soccer, lacrosse, hockey, rugby, and volleyball. This exercise will assist you greatly in turning, doing crossover steps, completing a push-off, and in shifting your weight from one leg to the other. In addition, the adductors are very important in swimming (especially the breast stroke) and in soccer when kicking with the inside of the foot (side passes). Development of these muscles is also important in bodybuilding to increase the size of the thighs and to maintain strong hip joints.

Execution

To isolate hip joint adduction and to keep the upper body motionless during execution, you should use a hip adductor machine such as the one made by Keiser. To position yourself, drop the back support of the machine so that you can lie flat with your body horizontal. Adjust the

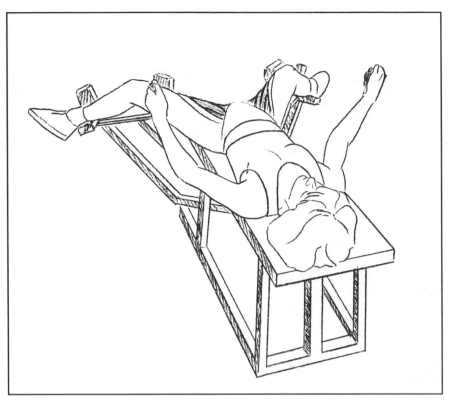

Figure 3.6
Muscles used in hip joint adduction

width of the leg units (how far apart you want the legs to be) by rotating the adjustment directly below the seat. Lie on your back and place your pelvis on the small seat so that it is directly above the axis of rotation of the machine. In this position your hip joint should line up with the axis of the machine. Place your leg in the resistance arm support and prepare to begin (see Photo 3.5).

When you are ready, inhale and hold your breath as you pull your thighs together. When your legs (thigh pads) touch (see Photo 3.6), exhale and relax your muscles somewhat to allow the legs to return to the initial apart position. Because of the eccentric return, keep your legs under control at all times.

Comments

• Do not set the adjustment so your legs are too far apart because this can cause injury, especially to the gracilis muscle, which is easily over-stretched. To prevent injury, and for overall safety when doing this exercise, you should start off with your legs apart at a comfortable position and then slowly increase the range of motion as you develop adequate strength and flexibility in the hip joint. Moving the legs apart as far as possible is important if you are a gymnast or a ballet dancer, but not for most individuals in their normal activities.

• I usually recommend that most people do this exercise while they are lying down on their back so that their body is in a relatively straight line. The reason for this is that when the muscles used in this exercise are used in sports or other activities, this is the position that the body is in. However, if this is not important to you, you can adjust the seat upward so that you are in more of a sitting position as you do this exercise.

• Strengthening the adductor muscles is very important for sports activities. However, it is not recommended that you use maximal weights and do few repetitions for two or three sets. The reason for this is that overdevelopment of these muscles may create excessive hypertrophy and, as a result, chafing of the

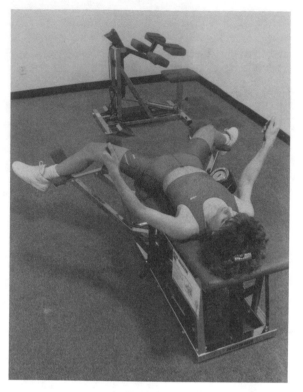

Photo 3.5

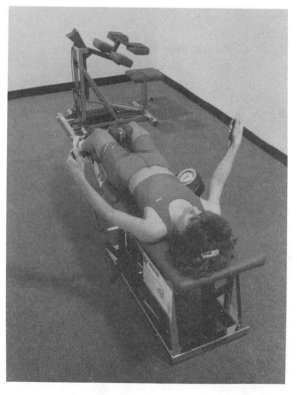

Photo 3.6

thighs when you walk or run. Thus, for most individuals, higher repetitions are usually recommended. Moreover, athletes must do this exercise for strength as well as for strength endurance, and this entails higher repetitions.

• When using the Keiser machine, you can adjust the resistance at any point in the range of motion. Thus, if you are in an extreme outward position, you may wish to decrease some of the resistance to prevent a muscle pull and increase it as you get closer to the midline. You can also increase the resistance on the return to work these muscles in the eccentric regime.

• For athletes I also recommend that they do some fast returns to develop more of the resiliency of these muscles as needed in many sports. In this case, do not go out to the extreme range but allow your legs to move apart approximately one-half to three-quarters the normal range and then quickly return them to the midline and repeat. These fast reversals in direction and muscular contraction are important for developing resiliency of the adductor muscles.

• For variety and also to improve your ability to do rotational cutting actions, you should do this exercise with your toes pointed inward and then with your toes pointed outward. Doing this helps to develop more of the rotational actions of these and other muscles.

• Hip adduction can also be done on a low pulley. In this variant you should keep your legs straight and start in the hip abducted position, that is, with the exercising leg away from the support leg. You then must keep the exercising leg straight and pull it down toward the support leg. However, because it is important to maintain an erect body position, you will have to hold onto the apparatus to maintain this position. Do not move your body from side to side during execution.

• When using the low pulley, many individuals like to bring the leg across the body in the belief that it works the muscles to a greater extent. However, this is not the case. When your leg crosses the midline, you must actually drop the pelvis on that side to allow the leg to cross over. Thus, instead of the hip adductors on the leg in motion being worked, you actually switch the action to the adductors of the support leg. Also, if you do high repetitions in this manner, because the pelvis is in motion and is attached to the spine, a tremendous lateral flexion of the spine is created, which can cause injury.

■ Hip Joint Abduction

Hip abduction is very important for athletes because it is the key action for lateral movement. In addition, the gluteus medius, which is involved in hip abduction, is the main muscle involved in holding the pelvis level while a person is running. Hip abduction is also a key exercise for bodybuilding. The best hip abduction exercise is performed on an exercise machine such as the one made by Keiser.

Major muscles and actions involved

The major muscle involved in thigh abduction is the gluteus medius. Some anatomists believe that the gluteus minimus is also a prime mover (see Figure 3.7). In this exercise the legs are pushed out to the sides of the body (away from the midline).

Sports uses

The gluteus medius and leg abduction are used in all sports requiring side stepping or movement to the side (lateral movement). This includes soccer, baseball, football, lacrosse, field and ice hockey, handball, basketball, volleyball, and racquet sports such as tennis and racquetball. Leg abduction is also the key action in shifting your body weight in the hitting and throwing sports. This occurs when you push off your rear leg to get your body weight onto your forward leg. Thus it is needed in baseball batting, the golf swing, tennis forehands and backhands, baseball pitching, football passing, the shot put, and discus and javelin throws.

In addition, the gluteus medius plays an important role in walking and running by keeping the pelvis level. When the muscle is weak, your

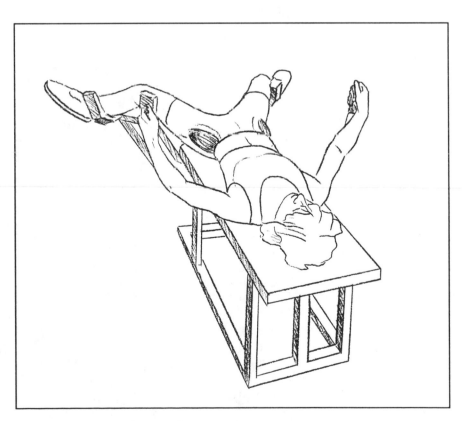

Figure 3.7
Muscles used in hip joint abduction

hips will drop on the side of the swing leg and in time this can cause back problems. Body-builders need the muscle development for shapely sides of the hips.

Execution

Hip abduction is best executed on a exercise machine, especially the one made by Keiser. To properly position yourself, put the back support down so that you are lying down in a horizontal position when you place your legs inside the padded leg resistance levers. In this position your body should basically be in a straight line. Position your pelvis on the little seat so that the axis of the hip joint is directly above the axis of rotation in the machine. Hold onto the grips with your hands to stabilize your upper body and to change resistance according to your abilities (see Photo 3.7).

When you are ready, inhale slightly more than usual and hold your breath as you pull your legs apart as far as possible (see Photo 3.8). Keep your toes pointed upward during the outward action. For most people the range of motion will be between 30 and 60 degrees on each side of the midline. Exhale and relax the muscles slightly as you return your legs to the initial together position.

Comments

- It is very important that your body remain in a straight line during execution of this exercise. When you raise the back support so that you are in more of a seated position, the gluteus medius ends up in a curved position from origin to insertion. Thus, when you do multiple repetitions you can irritate the joint, which in time can cause injury. It should also be noted that when your body is in a relatively straight position, it duplicates more closely the actions used in normal everyday activities like running, jumping, lateral movement, walking, and so on.
- When using the Keiser hip abductor machine, the exercise can be done in a fast and explosive manner to duplicate more closely the actions used in sports. To perform the exercise in this manner, as your legs come together, quickly reverse the action and pull them apart. The range of motion is not maximal in this case so that the muscles are not over-stretched. When

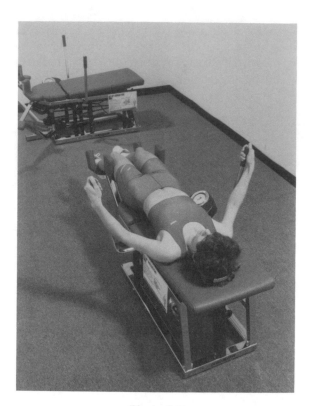

Photo 3.7

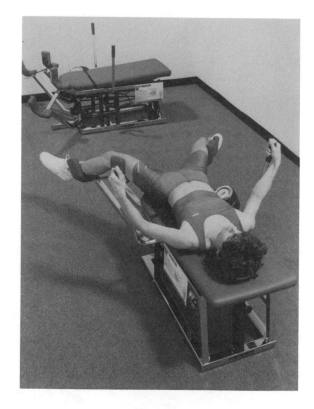

Photo 3.8

the exercise is performed like this, the hip abductor muscles are placed on stretch on the return, especially because of the strong eccentric return, and then switched to the concentric as the legs are pulled apart. This helps develop resiliency in these very important muscles. These actions cannot be done on other leg abductor machines because of the momentum generated by the weight stacks. If needed, abduction can be done with one leg in a fast or slow manner.

- Hip abduction can also be done on a pulley machine. To do so, you must stand sideways to a low pulley with the leg to be exercised farthest from the pulley. Begin the exercise with your legs together for a full range of motion. Keep the exercising leg straight and pull the cable away from your body. When doing this exercise, it is important that you keep your upper body erect at all times. Many people have a tendency to lean away from the direction that the leg is moving to create the range of motion. However, in doing so, the abductor muscles on the moving leg are not being worked. Note that on the Keiser machine you can hold your body in place so no lateral movement occurs.

- Many individuals have a tendency to point their toes outward in order to increase the range of motion. However, when you do this you actually must rotate your pelvic girdle backwards so that, in essence, you are doing more hip flexion than hip abduction. This is why it is important to keep your toes pointed directly in line with your legs. This problem does not arise when using the abductor machines because the legs and upper body are firmly stabilized with the machine, so the pelvis cannot be rotated. Thus, when using the leg abductor machine, you can turn your toes slightly inward or outward to develop more of the medial and lateral rotation actions. These actions are very important in almost all sports when you twist and turn your trunk when your leg is in contact with the floor.

- The Keiser hip abductor machine is also very effective when you are recovering from injury because you can adjust and change the amount of resistance at any point in the range of motion to accommodate your strengths and weaknesses. In this way you can continue to exercise in a safe manner.

■ The Good Morning

Bending forward with a rounded spine, especially when you are holding weights in your hands or on your shoulder or when you are trying to lift an object off the floor can be very dangerous. To learn how to bend correctly from your hips and to maintain your spine in its normal slightly arched position, you should do the good morning.

Major muscles and actions involved

The gluteus maximus and the upper hamstrings are involved in hip joint extension, while the erector spinae is involved in statically holding the spine in proper alignment (see Figure 3.8, muscles used in the deadlift). In this exercise the trunk is raised up and back from a forward lean position with the axis of rotation in the hips.

Sports uses

The muscles and actions involved in the good morning are needed in football (linemen coming off the line), weightlifting (clean and snatch and clean and jerk), and in powerlifting (deadlift). To a lesser extent the exercise is useful for running (the push-off phase), baseball and softball fielding, jumping, gymnastics, diving and trampolining (hip action), and in wrestling in various moves.

This exercise is also very important in bodybuilding for shape and definition of the buttocks, upper thighs, and lower back. Also, it is valuable in all lifting activities, especially when the weight is fairly heavy.

Execution

Stand upright with a barbell on your shoulders or dumbbells in your hands. Your feet should be approximately shoulder-width apart and your hands wider apart to hold the barbell. Your knees should be slightly bent for better balance, and the lumbar area of your spine should be in its normal alignment, that is, with a slight arch, at all times (see Photo 3.9). When you are ready, inhale slightly more than usual and hold your breath as you bend forward from your hip joints. Push your hips backward as your trunk comes forward and down to the horizontal position (see Photo 3.10) and then reverse directions and rise up to the starting position. Exhale as you approach the upright position.

Comments

- The major workload in execution of this exercise falls on the hip joint extensors, the gluteus maximus, and the hamstrings. These are big, strong muscles! Do not lift with your back (spine) muscles. They contract isometrically to hold the spine in place (in its arched position) and do not allow any movement. However, it should be noted that the isometric contraction (although not as effective as the concentric contraction) strengthens the spinal muscles. Thus, the entire back side is strengthened as a unit.

- In the early stages of doing this exercise, use light weights (or no weights) and execute the exercise slowly. This allows you to learn and become accustomed to the exercise more effectively. When you can perform the exercise correctly, gradually increase the weights but still keep them within your capabilities.

- As an advanced exercise the good morning is done with the legs kept straight, and to do so, considerable hip joint flexibility and balance are needed. Also, you must have well-developed spinal and hip joint extensor muscles. Do not execute this exercise in this manner until you meet these conditions.

- It should also be noted that the good morning is an excellent exercise for stretching the hamstrings. The usual sit and reach or standing toe touch (which are touted as the best hamstring stretches) actually stretch the spine more than the hamstrings. For example, in the standing toe touch, when you incline your trunk forward in a relaxed state, the erector spinae muscles contract eccentrically to control the downward motion but only for approximately 45 degrees. When you drop your trunk lower, the muscles are no longer holding the spine in place and thus you are literally hanging by the ligaments. You must stretch the ligaments tremendously to place your hands on the floor. This is an extreme example of flexibility, far past the normal range of motion in the waist.

  However, if you need this type of flexibility, as required in some sports such as gymnastics and diving, then you must do back raises and other exercises to strengthen your lower back. If this is not done, you will be highly prone to injury and back problems in later years. It is important to understand that flexibility is very important, but it should not go beyond the

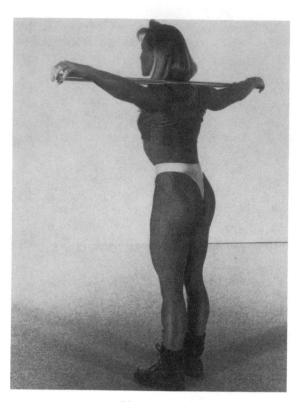

Photo 3.9

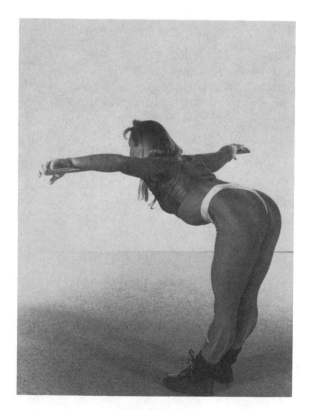

Photo 3.10

normal range. When it does, the ligaments become stretched, which creates a looser joint, making you more susceptible to injury.

The good morning produces the opposite effect—a stronger back and greater hamstring flexibility. In addition, the hamstrings and gluteus maximus are strengthened. Because of this, the good morning should be done by most athletes and fitness buffs as a prerequisite to the squat, deadlift, lunge, leg press, and glute-ham-gastroc raise.

■ Deadlift

The deadlift is one of the most negatively criticized exercises used by bodybuilders and athletes. And for good reason. When done incorrectly, the deadlift (bent knee or straight leg) can be very dangerous to the spine. However, when done correctly it is an excellent exercise for development of the buttocks, hamstrings, and, to a good extent, the lower back and anterior thighs.

Major muscles and actions involved

In this exercise the gluteus maximus and the upper hamstrings are involved in hip joint extension, and the erector spinae is involved in statically holding the spine in lordosis, that is, slightly arched in the lower spine (see Figure 3.8). In the bent-leg version the quadriceps femoris muscle group is also involved in knee joint extension . Execution of this exercise involves raising your trunk (and a barbell on the floor) from a forward bent-over position to a fully erect position.

Sports uses

Because the muscles and actions are identical to the squat (bent-knee variant) and the good morning (straight-leg variant), the sports uses are the same as for those two exercises.

Execution

Stand close to a barbell on the floor and bend over from your hips as in the good morning exercise and then bend your knees until you can grasp the barbell. When in position, your back should be in lordosis, and your trunk at approximately a 45-degree angle above the hori-

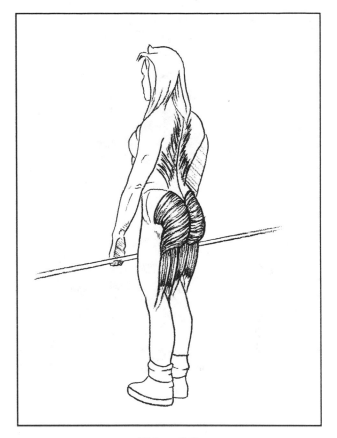

Figure 3.8
Muscles used in the deadlift

zontal. Keep your arms straight and grasp the bar with a slightly wider than shoulder-width grip (see Photo 3.11). Use a pronated (overhand) grip if the weights are light and a mixed grip (one hand pronated, one hand supinated) when the weights are heavy.

When you are ready, inhale and hold your breath as you raise your body and the barbell with knee and hip joint extension. Keep the weight equally distributed on both your feet. Keep pulling the barbell with a leg push and then with hip joint extension until you assume an erect body position with your chest out and your shoulders back (see Photo 3.12). Your arms should also pull from the shoulders but remain straight throughout the lift. Also, keep your spine arched throughout the entire movement. As you reach the ending position, exhale and relax slightly. When you are ready to return the bar to the bottom position, inhale and hold your breath to control your body as you reverse the actions to lower the barbell. If the barbell is not placed

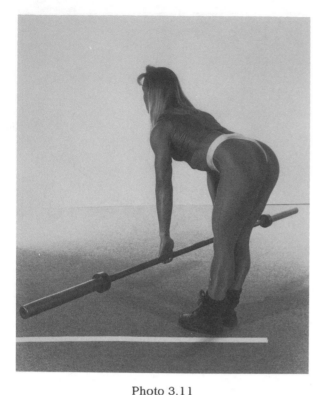

Photo 3.11

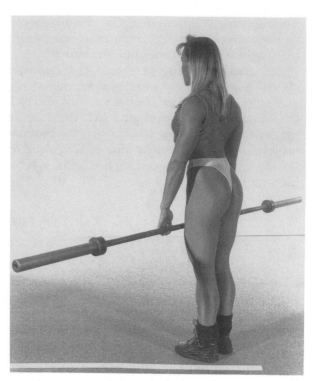
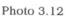

Photo 3.12

on the floor, keep holding your breath until you pass the most difficult part of the up phase and then exhale.

Comments

- The deadlift is very similar to the squat in many respects. The knee and hip action is basically the same, with the only major difference being the position of the barbell and your trunk. In the deadlift your trunk is inclined forward more and the weight is farther from the body. Regardless of these differences, the squat is a very effective supplementary exercise to assist in doing the deadlift.
- When using heavy weights it is usually not advisable to use wrist straps to hold the barbell because the use of straps may eventually weaken your fingers. If you are unable to hold the barbell with a reverse grip, do finger flexion exercises to strengthen your grip (see finger flexion in Chapter 11).
- For proper and safe execution of the deadlift, you must have a strong lower back. Your spine must be held in lordosis throughout the exercise to prevent any rounding movement of the spine. In addition to allowing you to do the

exercise correctly, a rigid spine allows you to do it safely. If you have a weak back or cannot hold your back in an arched position all the time, you should do back raises and good mornings for strengthening.

- You can do a stiff-leg deadlift, but only if you have great hamstring flexibility and a strong back. If you do not have the necessary flexibility and strength, you will have to bend your spine to reach the weight. Lifting in this position can be very dangerous to the lumbar spine. When pulling with your back rounded, you not only strain the erector spinae muscles greatly, but you also strain the ligaments. Keep in mind that when the back is rounded as you bend forward, the forces involved are doubled or tripled very quickly. Because of this, you should not do the stiff-leg (or the regular) deadlift with a rounded back.

  In view of this information, it is amazing to see many athletes and bodybuilders trying for a greater range of motion when doing the deadlift. Some even stand on a bench so that the weights can drop below the level of the bench when they do the exercise. However, in going through such an extreme range of motion, the back is rounded and, in time, these athletes develop injuries.

What is even more amazing is that this type of flexibility is not needed in nearly any sport, and it does not create greater strength of the muscles involved because the major load falls on the ligaments. If you need this range of motion, do the good morning until you can lower your head and shoulders (with the spine arched) down to about knee level. Then you will have the prerequisite hip joint and back strength to do the stiff-leg deadlift through a maximum range.

4 Combination Exercises

There are several excellent exercises that involve the hip joint and knee joint simultaneously or in sequence. These exercises are called combination or multi-joint exercises. The more effective ones will be described.

■ Squat

The squat has long been considered the king of exercises, and for good reason. It is a very effective exercise for developing the front and back sides of the thighs as well as the buttocks and, to a limited extent, the lower back. However, many people have been injured doing the squat, and as a result, it is not as popular as it once was. Thus, how you do the squat in relation to your abilities is crucial.

Major muscles and actions involved

Extension occurs in the knee joint as the thigh moves away from the shin as the leg straightens. The major muscle involved is the quadriceps femoris group. In the hip joint, extension occurs as the thigh moves up and forward to be in line with the upper body. The major muscles involved are the gluteus maximus and the hamstring muscle group. The ankle joint is also involved, but it is mostly passive. The erector spinae muscles contract isometrically to stabilize the spine (see Figure 4.1).

Sports uses

Knee and hip joint extension and the muscles involved are very important in execution of basic skills such as jumping for height or distance, all forms of running, various kicking actions, skipping, leaping, lifting, and pushing with the lower body. The sequential and combined knee and hip joint actions make these movements possible.

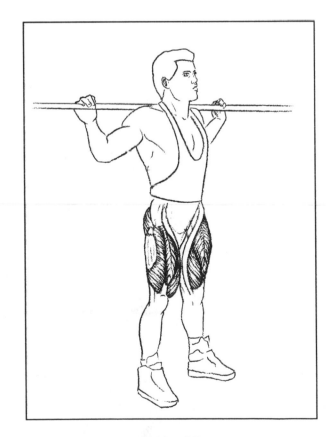

Figure 4.1
Muscles used in the squat

More specifically, these actions are needed in the high jump, basketball rebounding and shooting, blocking and spiking in volleyball, running and standing long jumps, bounding, squat jumps, kicking in karate and other martial arts, rugby, football, and soccer. They are also important in boxing for up to 30 percent of the total force delivered. In all sports that require running, hip joint extension is the main action which propels the runner forward immediately on touchdown, whereas knee joint extension is needed at the end of the push-off.

Without hip and knee joint extension, it would be impossible to lift weights off the floor. These actions are especially needed in the deadlift and squat events in the sport of powerlifting and in the clean, snatch, and clean and jerk exercises in weightlifting. Bodybuilders need these actions and the respective muscles to develop and define the anterior thigh and buttocks muscles. Also, the isometric contraction of the erector spinae strengthens the back, and a stronger back is a deterrent to injury and allows the lower body forces to be transferred to the upper body safely.

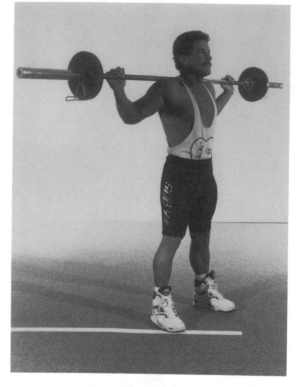

Photo 4.1

Execution

Stand up with your feet placed approximately shoulder-width apart and your toes pointed straight ahead or turned outward slightly. Hold a barbell behind your neck across your shoulders and resting on your upper trapezius muscle. Your grip should be a little wider than shoulder-width apart, but you can vary this grip if it does not feel comfortable for you. Your body weight should be equally distributed between both your feet (see Photo 4.1).

Inhale and hold your breath as you flex your knees and slowly lower your body into the squat position. Keep your heels in contact with the floor at all times and concentrate on lowering your hips. Your knees should come forward slightly, your buttocks should move slightly to the rear and then straight down, and your trunk should incline forward (up to 45 degrees from the vertical). Keep your spine arched in its normal position all the way to the bottom position, in which your thighs should be approximately horizontal. Your eyes should be focused directly in front of you (see Photo 4.2).

As you reach the bottom position, keep holding your breath as you quickly reverse directions by forcefully extending (straightening) your legs

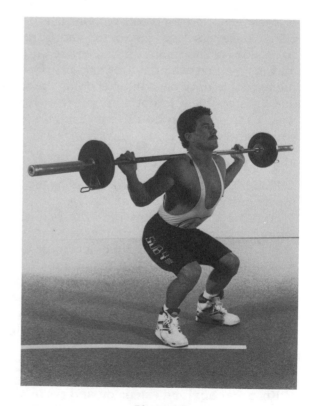

Photo 4.2

via hip and knee joint extension. (Hip extension is most important here.) Be sure your lower back remains arched in the down position and as you rise up. As you pass the sticking point as you are rising up, begin to exhale and complete the exhalation when you are in a full standing position. If very heavy weights are used and you experience difficulty as you come up, you can purse your lips and release very small amounts of air through them to relieve some of the pressure.

Comments

- The depth of the squat has been a matter of discussion for many years. Many doctors advise against going into a deep squat in the belief that it can hurt the knees. World-class weightlifters, however, go into extremely deep squats in which their buttocks almost touch the floor. From all indications, they do not suffer from bad knees any more than bodybuilders or powerlifters do. The key to doing the squat properly is to keep your heels on the floor so that your knees are over your feet. Raising your heels will cause your knees to move forward outside the support base, which places additional stress on the knees.

  If you find that your heels keep coming up when you squat, the problem is usually a lack of flexibility, especially in the Achilles tendon and hamstring muscles. To improve the flexibility of the hamstrings without weakening them, you should do good morning exercises (described in Chapter 3) using no weight. The good morning exercise will also strengthen your lower back and accustom it to being arched at all times as it is while doing the squat. If you still have problems after successfully doing the good morning exercise, then you should also do calf stretches to give you the necessary ankle joint flexibility.

- For proper and safe execution of the leg squat, you must have a strong lower back to prevent buckling or any undesirable movement of the spine. It should again be stressed that the spine must remain in its normal lordotic (arched) position throughout the entire movement. This is especially important in the bottom position. To check to see if your back is properly arched, look at yourself from the side in a mirror when you are in the bottom position; you should see an arch.

Too often bodybuilders and athletes allow their hips to roll under in the bottom position either because of a weak back or poor flexibility. But it is this rounding of the spine that causes injury. When your spine is rounded, excessive stress is placed on the anterior aspects of the vertebrae and discs and the weight is not equally distributed throughout the spine. If your lower back muscles are not strong enough to execute the squat properly, you should strengthen them by performing back raises and back raises with a twist (see Chapter 6).

To maintain the arch in your lower back, you must hold your breath during execution of the exercise. If you exhale either on the way down or on the way up, the intra-abdominal and intrathoracic pressure will decrease. When this happens you will not have the necessary rigidity to hold your spine in place. In essence, you need a partial Valsalva maneuver (an elevated pressure in the abdominal and thoracic cavities) to ensure safety to the spine when executing this exercise.

- It is also important that you look directly ahead during the entire execution of the exercise. Some people look at the ceiling as they do this exercise in order to keep their back arched. However, when you do this you lose perspective of your body's position. You must have some orientation to your surroundings for stability, which is very important in this exercise. Also, if you have sufficient strength in your lower back and flexibility in your hip joints, you will be able to hold the arch in your back without having to place the stress on your neck when you look upward.

- For greater variety and to place greater stress on the knees, you can perform the front squat exercise. To execute, place the barbell high on your chest so that it rests across your shoulders on the deltoid muscles. Hold your elbows high throughout the movement to prevent the bar from rolling off. For ease in holding the barbell, you can cross your forearms and support your hands on your shoulders.

  The front squat requires less balance than the back squat because your trunk remains in a more upright position throughout the movement. As in the back squat, however, be sure that your weight remains equally distributed on your whole foot because if the weight shifts onto the balls or heels of your feet, even greater pressure will be placed on your knees.

• The squat should be executed in one basic pattern. However, there are several variants that can be used for maximum all-around development. For example, use a narrow stance and a wide stance and do the exercise with your toes pointed straight ahead or outward. Do not point your toes inward because if you do so, when you go down into the squat, shearing forces will be created in the knee that can cause severe injuries (although it's perfectly safe to point your toes in when you are standing up).

Pointing the toes out is safe in the standing and squatting positions, because when the toes are pointed out, the knee also rotates outward so that there is no twisting in the knee joint during the up and down motion. However, pointing your toes out and then lowering yourself and bringing your knees inward can cause severe rotation in the knee, which can also cause injury. Always be sure that your leg remains in its normal anatomical position, that is, with the knee pointed to the front when the toes are pointed straight ahead and the knee pointed outward when the toes are pointed outward.

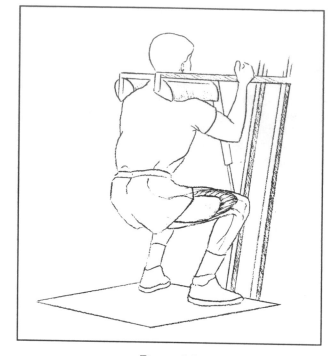

Figure 4.2
Muscles used in the machine squat

■ Machine Squat

For variety, or if you have trouble doing the squat correctly without pain or discomfort, you should use a squat machine. For effective execution you can use a Smith machine and do a half-squat, or you can do the exercise on a machine such as the one by Keiser, which allows you to add even more variety to the exercise (see Figure 4.2). Basic execution is the same for all variants.

Major muscles and actions involved

These are the same as in the squat.

Sports uses

The same as for the squat.

Execution

Because of its greater versatility, execution on the Keiser squat machine will be described. To begin, adjust the range of motion for the squat

by inserting a pin in the correct position on the limiting rod (similar to placing rods in a power rack [squat rack]). To position yourself properly, you must go into a semi-squat to get your shoulders under the resistance lever arm pads. Then extend your legs while keeping your back in its normal arched position and move to an upright standing position. Your feet should be placed slightly ahead of your shoulders, depending upon your flexibility and comfort level (usually 6–10 inches). Note that this is different than in a normal squat in which your feet are directly under your shoulders in the initial position. Adjust the resistance on the hand grip finger controls (see Photo 4.3).

When you are in position, adjust the air to the necessary resistance. When you are ready, inhale and hold your breath as you lower your body into the squat. Keep your spine in its normal anatomical position and fairly vertical. Lower your body until your thighs are parallel to the floor and there is a 90-degree angle between your trunk and thigh and between your shin and thigh (see Photo 4.4). Keep holding your breath as you quickly reverse the downward motion and rise up to the standing position.

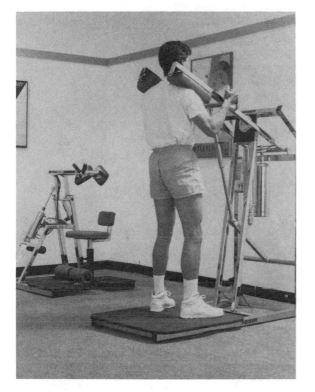

Photo 4.3

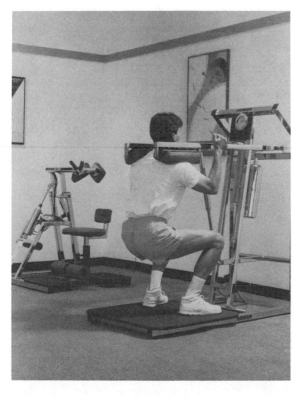

Photo 4.4

Comments

- In execution of this exercise be aware that your spine should remain in a fairly vertical plane at all times and the normal arch should be maintained in your lower back. In this variant there is little forward inclination of the back, and as a result, you will have less of a tendency to round your back in the bottom position as you do when executing the regular squat. Thus, be sure that your feet are in front of your center of gravity in the initial position. You must be very, very flexible and strong in the hip, knee, and ankle joints to place your feet farther under your body.
- It is important not to speed up in the downward movement. You should resist the eccentric return on the Keiser machine and quickly reverse direction in the bottom position. Doing this helps to build the resiliency of the knee muscles, which are most important in the running and jumping sports as well as in weightlifting. If you accelerate in the downward motion, the eccentric contraction cannot stop you and you must then rely on your knee ligaments to slow you, and these can easily be injured if the forces are great enough.

  When you maintain a steady slow to moderate downward speed, the eccentric contraction will actually slow you down as you approach the bottom position so that it is easier to reverse the direction quickly. If you go down to the bottom position and hold, you will lose some of the tension of the eccentric contraction and therefore have less force to raise you back up.

  If you use a Keiser machine, you should decrease the resistance and then you can return without any problems. However, on other machines (such as the Smith machine or the hack squat) this is not possible. Thus you must be extra careful when using these machines or have spotters available.
- For greater strength gains when using the Keiser squat machine, you can adjust the resistance so that you perform a combination of isometric, eccentric, and concentric contractions during the exercise. Studies have shown that doing a combination of all three muscle contraction regimes is more effective than doing only the common concentric contraction (which occurs in the up phase).
- For example, you can increase the resistance and slowly lower yourself into the squat to get

an overload in the eccentric muscle regime. It should be noted that this exercise is very effective for athletes because it is the eccentric contraction that stops the downward motion in jumping and running and creates the tension needed for the push-off in both events. You can also do this exercise by increasing the resistance close to the sticking point so that you can do isometrics to help overcome this difficult point. Or, you can increase the resistance at any point in the range of motion to get the specific development needed.

• Also very important is that you can change the resistance during execution of the exercise. Thus, you can increase or decrease the resistance on either the way up or the way down. No other machine has this interactive feature. In most machines you must adjust to the machine movements. With the Keiser machine, you make the machine adjust to your abilities.

• The Keiser squat machine also makes it possible to do the single-leg squat exercise, which is very difficult to execute with free weights because of the need for greater balance. But the single-leg squat is a very important exercise to develop strength and explosiveness. Most sports activities, including jumping and running, require a push-off with one leg rather than with two. Thus, when you do the single-leg squat, you can more closely duplicate the actions used in running or jumping. Also, a single-leg squat is less dangerous than a double-leg squat because less resistance compresses the spine. Moreover, a single-leg squat will produce the same amount of work on one leg with half the resistance needed for a double-leg squat.

• It is also possible to do a variant of the lunge. To execute this, do a single-leg squat, extending your free leg to the rear as you do so. Very advanced performers can also do both the single-leg squat and the lunge with the Strength Shoe on the Keiser Machine

• The Keiser squat machine can be used to perform this exercise quickly. When using the machine, you should drop down through a short range of motion and immediately leap up. Because of the strong eccentric pressure that is placed on your shoulders, you will not leave the floor. When doing this variation, you should not do a full squat. This exercise is used to duplicate the action used in running and

jumping in which the knee goes through only approximately 20–30 degrees of motion.

■ Strength Shoe Squat

For greater variety and to work the calf muscles, a good exercise is the squat done while you wear Strength Shoes. This is an advanced exercise and is not recommended for beginners because of the stress needed to maintain proper body position.

Major muscles and actions involved

In the knee and hip joints the muscles and actions are the same as in a free weight or machine squat. However, with the Strength Shoe you also bring in dynamic action of the ankle joint to keep your feet flat. (Because the Strength Shoe has a platform under the ball of the foot area, the heel is free to move.) Thus, there may be some dynamic and isometric ankle joint flexion and extension, which involves the soleus and gastrocnemius muscles (see Figure 4.3).

Sports uses

The same as for the squat.

Execution

Execution is basically the same as in the free weight squat (see Photos 4.5 and 4.6). However, when you wear Strength Shoes, you must pay attention to maintaining your foot position and body balance. In addition, you should adhere to all of the recommendations given for the proper execution of the free weight squat.

Comments

• When you do this exercise with Strength Shoes, the base area is much smaller (only the front part of the foot). Therefore, many muscles, including the midsection muscles, must contract more strongly to help you maintain your balance. Because of this, there is greater involvement and more development of these muscles, especially in regard to their stabilizing actions. In addition, the calf muscles are greatly involved in helping to give you stability, and therefore these muscles are developed. The calf muscles are not involved in the other variants of the squat because your feet remain flat on the floor while you do them.

- Because of the greater stability needed to do this variant, you should not use a great deal of weight. Initially, start with only your body weight and gradually increase the resistance as you are able to maintain your position.

- When you are accustomed to doing the exercise at a slow to moderate rate of speed, you can alter the exercise slightly. To do so, decrease the depth of the squat by one-half and lower yourself at a slightly faster rate. As soon as you reach the bottom position, quickly reverse the direction of movement and rise up quickly. You should slow down and stop by the time your body is straight, with your feet still in contact with the floor. Doing this produces slightly greater action in the ankle joint so that you involve the calf muscles in a more dynamic and resilient manner. In addition, this enables the knee and hip joint muscles to react in a resilient manner, which is very important in jumping and running activities. This is the basis for explosiveness, which underlies all speed movements.

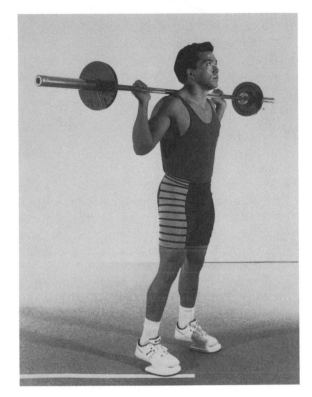

Photo 4.5

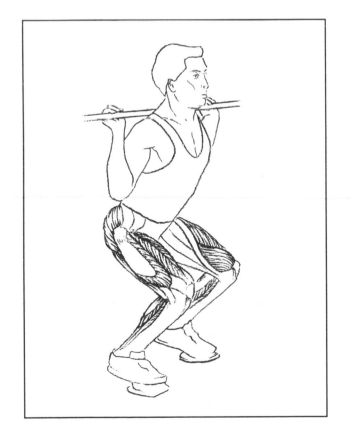

Figure 4.3
Muscles used in the Strength Shoe squat

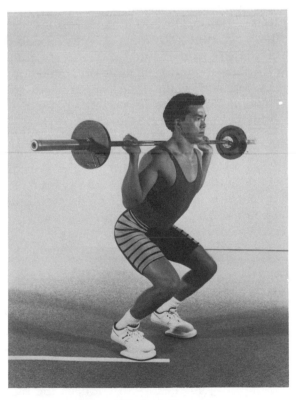

Photo 4.6

- Because the Strength Shoes provide no support for your heels, when you do walking and running actions when wearing the shoes, your heel travels through a greater range of motion. This helps to stretch the Achilles tendon and to increase the range of motion in the ankle, which will help you increase your speed and jump height. In essence, the shoes allow you to duplicate the exact muscular contractions used in explosive sports.
- Because of their effectiveness in developing muscle and tendon resiliency, Strength Shoes can also be worn as you perform plyometric exercises. These include various jumps on one or two legs, bounding squat jumps, split squat jumps, and side jumps. Be sure you have an adequate strength base before doing these activities. (For information on the Strength Shoe, call 1-800-451-JUMP).

■ Lunge

The squat is a very beneficial exercise, but it does not develop the legs and hips to as great an extent as is possible. To get a greater range of motion in the hip joint (greater stretch and contraction of the hip joint extensors) while at the same time creating a greater stretch of the hip flexors, you should do the lunge. This exercise is also quite effective and safe for knee development when done properly. Its greatest value, however, lies in stretching and strengthening the hip joint muscles.

Major muscles and actions involved

Extension occurs in the hip and knee joints. In this action the thigh moves away from the shin as the legs are straightened. In addition, the erector spinae muscles contract isometrically to stabilize the spine (see Figure 4.4).

Sports uses

With some minor exceptions, it can be said that the lunge is valuable in all the sports mentioned in the section on the squat exercise. However, the lunge also provides other benefits for sports, such as the development of hip joint flexibility, which is very important in running. In the push-off in running, the greater the flexibility of the hip joint flexors, the longer the push-off foot can remain in contact with the floor or

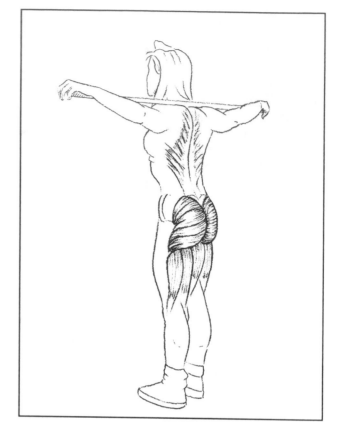

Figure 4.4
Muscles used in the lunge

ground and generate force to propel the body forward. When these muscles are tight, the runner has a tendency to push vertically rather than horizontally.

In addition, the lunge is very important in developing the maximum forward reaching action that is needed in the racquet sports. For example, to reach a ball far away from your body, you must step out and literally lunge for the ball. Thus, this action is important in basketball, in football tackling, in gymnastics for flexibility and strength of the muscles when going into a split, for maximum range of motion in splitting the legs in jumping in ballet and other types of dance, and in fencing.

Execution

Stand up and assume a well-balanced position as you hold a barbell across the front of your shoulders. Use a wider than shoulder-width grip and place your feet parallel to each other and between hip- and shoulder-width apart (see

Photo 4.7). When you are ready, inhale and hold your breath and step forward with a very long stride, keeping your back in a vertical, slightly arched position. Upon landing, hold the vertical position as you lower your trunk straight down.

At the bottom position, you should have approximately 90 degrees of flexion in your forward leg and most of the weight should be on it. Your rear leg should remain straight but relaxed (see Photo 4.8). You should feel tension in your front leg and lower back and a strong stretch of the hip flexors in the rear leg. When you have developed sufficient flexibility, your rear knee should touch the floor lightly in the bottom position. Once you have reached this lowermost position, shift the weight backward. As you do so, strongly extend your forward leg and take several short steps to return to the initial position. Exhale and repeat the exercise, stepping out with your other leg. This exercise should be done at a moderate speed and with a full range of motion.

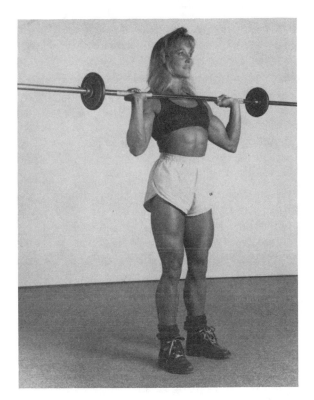

Photo 4.7

Comments

- In order to get the full benefits of this exercise in the hip joint area, it is essential that you keep your trunk erect. With your trunk in this position, there is maximum flexion in the hip joint of the forward leg in the down position. This, in turn, brings on a maximum stretch of the gluteus maximus muscle for a stronger contraction. In essence, the deeper the lunge, the greater the use of the gluteus maximus (and hamstrings) and the greater the hip joint flexibility.

  However, to get maximum flexibility in the hip joint of the forward leg, you must also have great flexibility in the hip joint of the rear leg. Most athletes feel a tremendous stretch on the hip flexors of the rear leg in the initial stages of this exercise. However, if you do the exercise slowly and gradually over a long period of time, you will develop the necessary flexibility to do the exercise for maximum effectiveness.

- This exercise can also be done effectively with the barbell held across the back of your shoulders (as in the back squat). With the barbell in this position you will have a greater tendency to lean your trunk forward, which may decrease the range of motion and the gluteus maximus muscle action. In addition, the spine can be injured if it is allowed to flex at the bottom position and if you have heavy weights

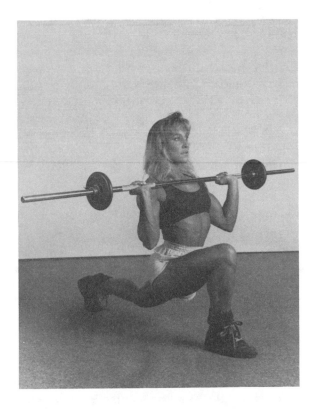

Photo 4.8

on your shoulders. (For proper execution with the bar on the back of the shoulders, see the Strength Shoe lunge.)

- Leaning forward is the most common error when doing the lunge. This is usually the result of poor hip joint flexibility and a weak lower back. Not only is leaning forward potentially injurious to the spine, but it places excessive pressure on the forward knee, which can also be damaging.

- When you contract the erector spinae strongly in order to hold your trunk erect, your pelvis is held in place (vertical) along with your trunk. Because of this, the lunge helps to develop the stabilizing actions of the erector spinae. Some people place their foot on a raised platform when they do the lunge, which allows them to lower their hips below the horizontal. This is done in an effort to get a greater range of motion in the hip joint, but, in reality, it defeats this purpose because when you lean forward, you allow your pelvic girdle to rotate forward. If you wish to do the lunge exercise this way, you can try it, although because of the extreme range of motion needed, it is usually reserved for gymnasts and dancers.

- The lunge and the glute-ham-gastroc raise (described later in the chapter) are used to a great extent by world class weightlifters to develop the hip and knee joint extensors. As mentioned earlier, these muscles and the quadriceps muscle of the knee joint are responsible for raising the bar off the platform. Only the hip joint extensors are especially important in raising the bar after it passes knee level. The lunge also develops the flexibility needed to go into a deep squat and the strength needed to rise out of a deep squat.

- The lunge exercise can also be done by rising up where your forward leg is placed (walking lunge). This action puts more tension on the knee joint extensors, and if great weights are used this exercise can cause injury to the knee joint because the knee is in an extreme forward position. Therefore, before rising, you should shift some of the weight backward until your shin is close to being vertical when you are rising up. Also, take a shorter stride when you are doing the walking lunge.

- The lunge can also be done to the side (see the section on the side lunge later in the chapter). This involves the adductors and abductors of the hip in addition to the hip and knee extensors.

- You can greatly increase your hip joint flexibility by doing long, deep lunges. If you have not done this exercise before, you should start by using light weights (or only your body weight) until you master the technique, and only then should you gradually increase the weights. Performing deep lunges with light weights will increase your flexibility and strengthen the tendons and ligaments of your hip and especially your knee joint. This will give you the prerequisites of strength and flexibility that you need in order to do the exercise using heavy weights. In this regard the lunge can be used as a prerequisite to doing the squat, especially the full-range squat.

If you have difficulty doing this exercise because of a lack of flexibility or balance, you should alter the method of execution. For example, after you step out and land, hold that position, keeping your trunk erect. Exhale somewhat and slowly lower your body to stretch your hip joint muscles gradually. Go as low as possible and hold the stretch for up to 10–20 seconds. Then inhale and hold your breath as you shift the weight back and push yourself back up to the initial position.

Because you exhale in the down position in this exercise, you should not use heavy weights. For most people, a light pole or bar held across the shoulders provides enough weight. However, if you are tight in the shoulders, use a pole such as the Exer-Stik which has a curved section so that it fits around your neck comfortably. This pole allows you to grip more effectively without any straining, which also makes it easier to move through the full range of motion.

■ Strength Shoe Lunge

One of the most troublesome areas for bodybuilders and athletes is the Achilles tendon and the calf muscles. The most effective exercises to work this area through a full range are the heel raise and the seated calf raise. However, the lunge exercise done while wearing Strength Shoes works this area very intensely through a lesser range.

Major muscles and actions involved

In the knee joint the major muscle is the quadriceps femoris muscle group (see Figure 4.5). In this action the thigh moves away from the shin as the legs straighten. Extension occurs in the hip joint, which involves the gluteus maximus and the upper portion of the hamstrings. In this action the thigh moves backward until it is in line with the pelvic girdle and upper trunk. In the ankle joint the major muscles involved are the gastrocnemius and the soleus. In addition, the Achilles tendon is also strongly involved. In this exercise the shin moves away from the foot in an action similar to pointing the toes. The erector spinae of the lower back stabilize the trunk in this exercise.

Sports uses

The movements and actions involved in this exercise are important in running sports and especially in sprinting because of the additional calf involvement. They are also important in all jumping activities in sports such as basketball, volleyball, track and field, soccer, and so on. In essence, the movements and actions in the Strength Shoe lunge are needed in almost all sports that involve resilient movement and the production of horizontal and vertical force. Thus, the lunging action is very important in the sports of tennis, racquetball, badminton, squash, table tennis, baseball, football, rugby, lacrosse, field and ice hockey, team handball, and handball.

The movements used in this exercise are also important in all the iron sports but especially in weightlifting (in executing the snatch and especially the clean and jerk). For bodybuilders, this exercise is very important for the development of the buttocks muscles, the upper posterior thigh, and the entire front of the thigh. Also, by using Strength Shoes you get effective development of the gastrocnemius and soleus (calf) muscles.

Execution

With a pair of Strength Shoes on your feet, stand up and assume a well-balanced position and hold the barbell on your shoulders behind your neck. Your weight should be on the balls of your feet (the platforms of the shoes) and your feet should be held in approximately their nor-

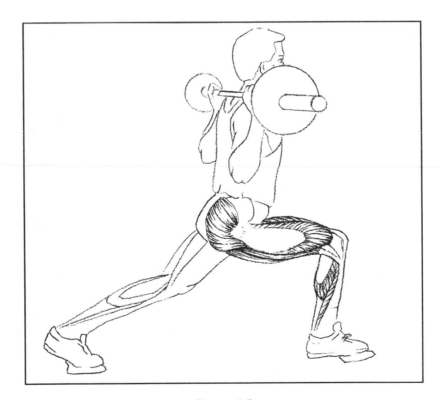

Figure 4.5
Muscles used in the Strength Shoe lunge

mal, anatomical position (your heel will be approximately 1½ inches off the floor so that your feet are level). Your feet should be parallel and between hip- and shoulder-width apart (see Photo 4.9).

When you are balanced and ready, take a very large step forward and plant your forward leg solidly on the support base of the shoe without letting your heel touch the floor. When you land, keep your trunk in an upright (vertical) position. When your body is stabilized, lower it until you feel a stretch in the hip flexors of your back leg and your forward leg hamstring and gluteus maximus muscles (see Photo 4.10). Your front leg should be at approximately a 90-degree angle (or slightly less) in the knee joint and bear almost all your body weight. Your rear leg should be straight but relaxed so that when you reach the bottom position (when you have developed considerable flexibility) your knee can touch the floor lightly.

After you reach the bottom position, strongly extend (plantar flex) your front foot to shift the weight backward and upward. As the weight moves backward, extend your front leg to raise your body and take two to three short steps until you are back at the original position. Repeat the exercise, stepping out with your other leg so that you alternate legs with each movement. When you are doing the exercise, concentrate on holding a good base, lowering your body for a full range of motion, and extending your foot and leg when you are rising up.

Your breathing must also be coordinated with these movements. As you start the exercise, inhale slightly more than usual and hold your breath as you do the lunge. Exhale after you extend your leg and as you return to the original position.

Comments

• In order to get the full benefits of this exercise in the hip joint area, it is essential that you keep your trunk erect. With your trunk in this position, there is greater use of the muscles involved and especially greater intensity of the calf muscle contraction. It should also be noted that the more you lower your body, the greater the stress, especially on your calves.

The reason the calves are more involved is that when you use the Strength Shoe, your calf muscles stretch and as a result produce a very strong eccentric contraction, which then al-

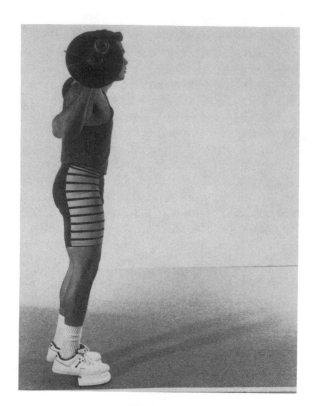

Photo 4.9

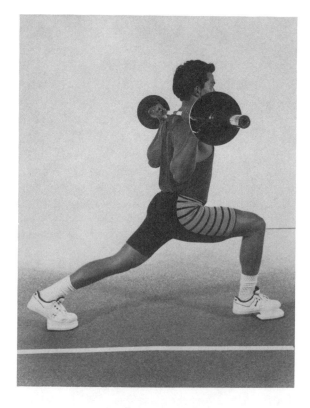

Photo 4.10

lows them to contract with even greater force when you rise up. Therefore, because of the greater intensity, you should alternate legs when doing this exercise so that your muscles have a chance to relax between repetitions. If you do not do this, your calf muscles can become very tight.

- In the usual one-step lunge movement in sports (as, for example, when you reach for a ball), you land heel first after you stride to ensure a longer reach. But when you have weights, this movement becomes dangerous— because of the greater resistance, landing on your heel does not allow for any cushioning or preparation of the muscles. Then when you land on the ground, the reaction forces travel up your leg and into your body, which can strain your hips, legs, or back. When you use Strength Shoes you should land on the ball of your foot (the platform under the front part of the foot). Because of the large surface area, your landing will be very stable, but you will have to contract your calf muscles strongly in order to hold your heel up. The energy accumulated in the gastrocnemius and soleus muscles is then returned in the push-off back to the initial position.

- Although this exercise involves strong work by the calf muscles, that does not mean that less work is done by the quadriceps or the gluteus and upper hamstring muscles. The only difference when using the Strength Shoes is that you get the added benefit of calf development.

- It is very important to breathe correctly when you do this exercise. You must hold your breath for a short period to stabilize your body when you touch down, especially if you are using fairly heavy weights. If you exhale at this time, your trunk may collapse and you will fall. Also, you must hold your breath on the push-off so that you can generate maximum force in your legs and keep your spine stable as you move yourself up and back.

- For maximum benefits, the lunge must be long. Keep in mind that the longer the lunge and the more you lower yourself, the greater the involvement of the hips, ankles, and knees. However, be sure that you can get up and move back from the forward position. Doing an extremely long lunge with weights and then not being able to return makes for a dangerous situation. Because of this, you must prepare yourself to do long lunges, especially with Strength Shoes. Gradually increase the distance and weights to build up to the final exercise.

- The lunge exercise can also be done by rising up at the place where your forward leg is placed. In this variant, commonly known as the walking lunge, you should take shorter strides. Also, this variant places more tension on the forward knee joint extensors and calf muscles. Thus, do not use great weights when you are doing the walking lunge. Performing this variant with Strength Shoes makes the exercise safer for the knees and also provides a greater range of muscle involvement.

■ Side Lunge

The lunge can also be done in a sideward direction with or without Strength Shoes. When doing a side lunge, the hip abductors and adductors are also involved in the exercise.

Major muscles and actions involved

These are the same as for the lunge. In addition, the gluteus medius is involved in hip abduction when you push out to the side, and the adductor longus, magnus, and brevis are involved in pulling your legs together in the upright position (see Figure 4.6). The calf muscles are also involved in maintaining your balance when you use Strength Shoes and in pushing off for the return.

Sports uses

The movement used in the side lunge is most useful for lateral movements and lateral movements done in combination with jumping for height or distance. It is used in different kinds of running as, for example, open field running in football, cutting actions, leaping to the side, pushing off in baseball pitching and batting, and other types of throwing and hitting. The combination of knee and hip joint extension together with abduction is also the major action involved in kicking as used in karate and other martial arts.

It should also be noted that this exercise will help you strengthen your hip and leg muscles, and will also help you develop greater flexibility in the inner thigh and groin area. This is very

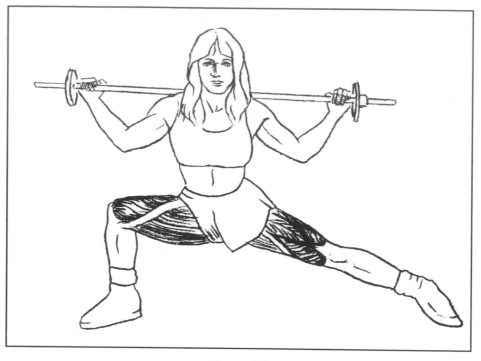

Figure 4.6
Muscles used in the side lunge

important in all sports that require lunging to the side or reaching actions.

Execution

Stand up and assume a well-balanced position with a barbell across your shoulders. Your feet should be parallel and wider than shoulder-width apart. Your trunk should be erect and you should use a wide grip on the barbell for better balance. When using Strength Shoes, keep your weight on the balls of your feet.

Push off to one side via hip abduction and step out with the leg on that side of your body. Turn your toes outward slightly so that when you land your leg is turned outward. Land on the ball of your foot, especially when you are using Strength Shoes. Then go into a squat on the lunging leg, keeping your trunk firm as you do so. Lower yourself until the thigh of your lunging leg is parallel to the floor and your push-off leg is relaxed but kept fairly straight at the knee joint (see Photos 4.11 and 4.12). Keep your head up and facing forward with your spine slightly arched throughout the movement. When you do this exercise with Strength Shoes, it is important to keep your heel off the floor at all times.

After the bottom position is reached, push yourself upward and sideward back to the initial position. Repeat the exercise, going to the opposite side. Speed of execution should be moderate with concentration on a full range of motion.

Comments

- When the lunge is done in one motion, you should inhale slightly more than usual and hold your breath as you execute the lunge and the return. Exhale after you pass the most difficult portion of the return and then assume the original position. Pause and then repeat with the opposite leg.
- To do the lunge to increase flexibility in your inner thigh, inhale slightly more than usual as you step out and land on the ground. Once you are securely in position, exhale and relax and gradually lower your body as you stretch your inner thigh. When you are ready to return to the original position, inhale again and hold your breath as you stand up and go back to the initial position.
- Because the side lunge can be a taxing exercise, especially if it is done with Strength Shoes on, you should be sure you have ample strength in

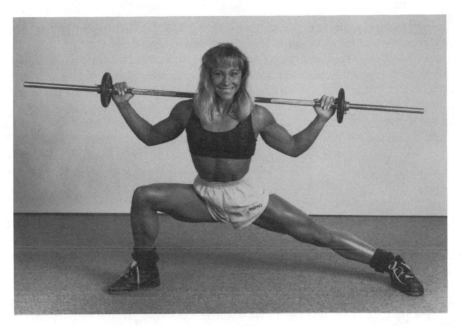

Photo 4.11

your knees and calf muscles before you do it. Because you are moving to the side, your knees must possess additional lateral strength which is not needed in exercises such as the squat and front lunge. It should also be noted that the hamstrings come into play to provide even greater lateral stability to the joint, especially if you use heavy weights.

- Strength is not the only physical quality needed for effective and productive execution of the side lunge. Total body balance and hip joint flexibility also play a major role. Because of this, you should not begin doing this exercise with heavy weights, even if you can handle them when you do the front lunge. Start with light weights and increase the weights only as you develop these physical qualities. You will know you are ready for heavier weights when you can go to the parallel thigh position and feel well-balanced with the other leg out to the side and straight.

- When you step out, be sure to point your toe slightly out to the side. In so doing, the action should occur in the hip joint, so that your knee is also lined up with your foot when you go into the squat portion of the lunge. If your toes are pointed forward and your knee is over the foot that faces sideways, great twisting forces can occur in the knee, and these can cause injury.

Also, the thigh of your push-off leg should be in the level position to ensure that the push-off action is via hip joint abduction and not extension, as in the front lunge.

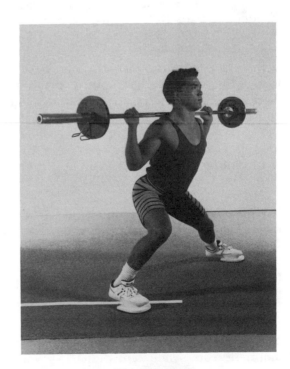

Photo 4.12

• When using Strength Shoes, the entire shoe platform should remain in contact with the floor in the down position. You will need a strong contraction of the gastrocnemius and soleus muscles to hold your heel up so that your foot remains parallel to the ground. Most individuals will experience a strong contraction in these muscles as they execute the exercise.

■ Leg Press

If you have a back, shoulder, or arm injury, doing the squat is very difficult, if not impossible. To eliminate these problems but still get very effective development of the same muscles, the leg press exercise can be done on a leg press machine (see Figure 4.7).

Major muscles and actions involved

The same as for the squat.

Sports uses

The same as for the squat.

Execution

To execute this exercise, a leg press machine must be used. Because of its greater versatility, the one made by Keiser will be described. However, the basic execution is the same for other leg press machines.

Sit down on the leg press machine so that your back is flush against the back support when your knees are bent at approximately a 90-degree angle measured between the back of the shin and the back of the thigh. After the seat is adjusted for this positioning, place both feet on the foot platforms, grasp the hand grips, and extend your legs. This is the starting position (see Photo 4.13).

When you are ready, adjust the air pressure for the necessary resistance with a press of your thumb as you hold onto the grips. (Note that on other machines you will have to set the resistance before you get into the machine.) Then inhale slightly more than usual and hold your breath as you bend your legs to allow the resistive foot platforms to move toward you. You will notice the foot platforms changing their angle of inclination in synchronization with your feet. (On some leg press machines, the foot platforms

are stationary and your body moves as a result of leg extension.)

As the angle in your knee joint approaches 90 degrees (see Photo 4.14), immediately push the foot platforms away until your legs are fully extended. At this point, exhale and relax momentarily before beginning the next repetition. On the Keiser as on most other machines, you will feel a strong return, so you must keep the movement under control. Hold the hand grips during execution, especially when more force is required.

Comments

• When you are doing this exercise, it is important that you go only to a 90-degree angle in the knee joint unless you have great flexibility and strength in your hip, knee, and ankle joints. With adequate flexibility you can let your knees come closer to your chest to place even greater stress on your hip joint extensors and knees. However, if you lack the needed flexibility and strength, bringing your knees up close to your chest will force your pelvic girdle to rotate backward, which will create a rounded spine. Doing this over a period of time can cause severe back problems.

• In executing the exercise with heavy weights, it is very important to control the weights as your knees approach your trunk. The gluteus maximus and quadriceps femoris muscle groups should undergo a strong eccentric contraction to control the resistance. You should make a fast change to concentric contraction at the end of the movement to help push the foot platforms back to the initial position. Such actions utilize the stored energy in the eccentric contraction. However, do not allow the foot platforms to come back too quickly because doing so can put excessive strain on your knee and hip joints, especially when you are going through a full range of motion.

You can do this exercise with quick, explosive-type movements on the Keiser machine. To do so, you should use a shortened range of motion and do the total movement very rapidly. You can continue the fast movements without having to stop. Done this way, this exercise more closely duplicates many sports actions, especially when it is done alternating your legs. However, keep in mind that such capabilities are not available on most other machines. On the Keiser machine you

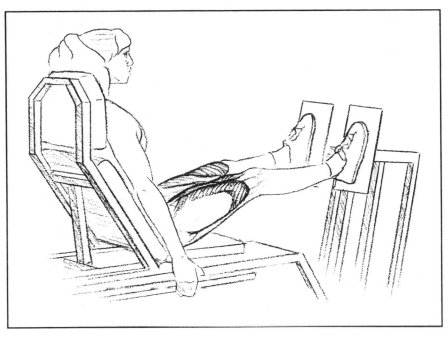

Figure 4.7
Muscles used in the leg press

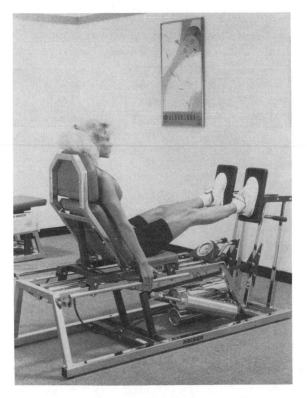

Photo 4.13

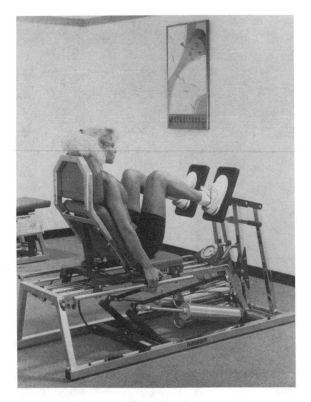

Photo 4.14

can also do one-leg presses, but only if you first shift your pelvic girdle to the outside so that your center of gravity is more in line with your foot placement.

■ Glute-Ham-Gastroc Raise

The name of this exercise is a very descriptive term that I coined to describe an exercise created by the Soviets to strengthen the gluteus maximus and total hamstring muscles. In the Soviet Union the exercise is done with a gymnastics horse and wall bars, but in the United States, because of the lack of such equipment, I created the Glute-Ham Developer on which to do this excellent exercise. It is the only exercise that develops the hamstring muscle from both ends in sequence. Athletes and bodybuilders using this exercise have found it amazingly effective for development of the hamstring muscles as well as for the prevention and treatment of hamstring injuries.

Major muscles and actions involved

In the hip joint the major muscles are the upper portion of the hamstring muscle and the gluteus maximus to perform hip joint extension (see Figure 4.8). In this action you raise your trunk, keeping it rigid, until it is in line with your legs. In the knee joint the major muscles are the lower hamstrings and the gastrocnemius muscle. They are involved in knee joint flexion, in which you raise your thigh (entire body) from the knee upwards while keeping your shin in place. Note that this is the opposite of what takes place in the knee curl.

Sports uses

The glute-ham-gastroc raise uses movements that are important in all sports that require lifting or rising up with a normally arched back such as weightlifting (cleans and rising out of the squat), powerlifting (squat, deadlift), football (linemen coming off the line), and baseball (fielding and catching overhead balls). These movements are also very important in all jumping activities, especially in jumping from a one-half to a deep crouch position. Examples of this include basketball (jumping for rebounds), volleyball (blocking and some spiking), the high jump, and the standing long jump.

This exercise is especially effective in developing the muscle movements used in all running activities, especially when the leg first contacts the ground in the paw-back action. In fact, the glute-ham-gastroc raise is very specific to this action. Thus, this exercise is important in baseball, football, basketball, track and field, soccer, lacrosse, rugby, hockey (ice and field), and so on. The glute-ham-gastroc raise is also very effective when used by bodybuilders because the total movement gives a much stronger "pump" to the hamstrings than can be achieved by the usual knee curl exercise.

Another very important use of the exercise is for the prevention of injuries to the hamstring muscles. Athletes who have done this exercise have reported the almost total absence of injuries to the hamstrings. In addition, they have found this exercise to be maximally effective in the rehabilitation of hamstring injuries.

Execution

This exercise is best executed on a BFS Glute-Ham Developer. To position yourself, assume a prone position on the apparatus and insert your feet between the rear padded rollers from the sides until your soles are against the back plate and your toes are pointed downward. The foot positioning unit should be adjusted so that the mid-portions of your thighs are in contact with the upper position of the rounded seat. Your knees should be 4–6 inches behind the back side of the seat. When your legs are in place, lower your trunk over and down the front portion of the seat so that your upper body and pelvic girdle form a straight line (vertical) from the hip joint to the floor. Cross your arms on your chest or behind your head for greater resistance (see Photo 4.15).

When you are in position, inhale slightly more than usual and hold your breath as you raise your trunk and pelvis with the axis in the hip joint. Your back should be kept rigid in its normal, slightly arched position at all times. After you raise your trunk so that your body forms a straight line from your head to your feet (see Photo 4.16), keep pulling with your hip joint extensor muscles and then bend your knees (knee joint flexion). Keep raising your body (from your knees to your head) until it is approximately 45 degrees above the horizontal (see Photo 4.17). After reaching this top position, exhale and relax slightly but keep your lower back in

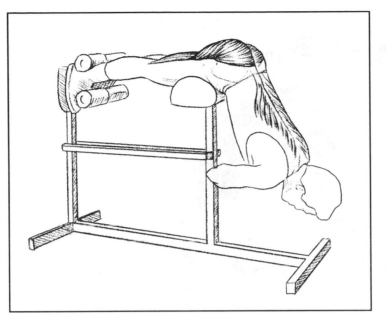

Figure 4.8
Muscles used in the glute-ham-gastroc raise

its arched position. Lower your body by straightening your legs and then flexing at the hip to return to the inverted position. Execute the exercise at a moderate rate of speed without any jerkiness, quick snaps, or fast changes in speed.

Comments

- This exercise can only be done on the Glute-Ham Developer or on a gymnastics horse with your feet between wall bars with the soles against the wall. Although the Glute-Ham Developer looks like a Roman chair, the Roman chair cannot be used for the execution of this exercise because it does not have a support for the soles of the feet or a bottom roller to secure the feet. In addition, and very importantly, the Roman chair cannot be adjusted for proper positioning, which is critical to safe and effective execution of this exercise. Therefore, to get the benefits described, do the exercise as described. Trying to do it any other way may lead to injury.
- From physiological studies, it is well known that two-joint muscles (such as the hamstrings) will contract most forcefully when only one end is in action (shortening). Simultaneous joint action at both ends of the muscle (when both ends of the muscle are being pulled to the belly of the muscle at the same time) will produce a weaker contraction. In the glute-ham-gastroc exercise the gluteus maximus and the upper end of the hamstrings contract initially to rotate your pelvic girdle backwards. In this action, these muscles raise your trunk when your spine is kept rigid by a strong isometric contraction of the erector spinae. When your trunk is in line with your legs, the upper hamstring goes into isometric contraction to hold this position since it is impossible to execute hip hyperextension.

After this, the lower end of the hamstrings and the upper gastrocnemius contract, creating knee joint flexion, which continues to raise your body, which should remain rigid. The contraction of the lower hamstrings occurs while the upper hamstrings are shortened and held under maximum tension, which results in a "super maximal" contraction of the entire muscle. In other words, at the end of the exercise, both the lower and upper portions of the hamstrings are in maximal contraction. Thus, in this exercise both ends of the hamstrings go into contraction in sequence, not simultaneously, to create maximum shortening. This is the main reason that the glute-ham-gastroc exercise is so effective for total hamstring development and the reason that this exercise is used very effectively in rehabilita-

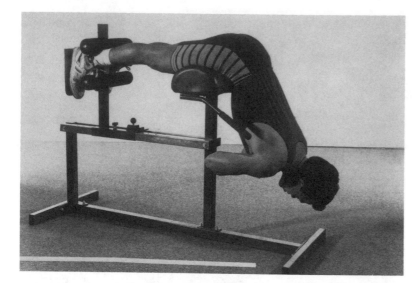

Photo 4.15

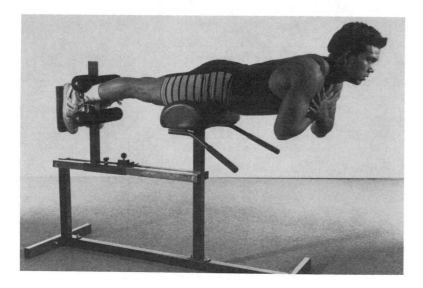

Photo 4.16

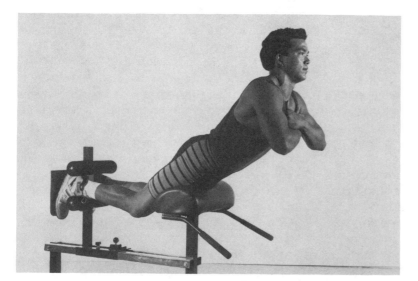

Photo 4.17

tion and for the prevention of hamstring injuries.

- Doing the glute-ham-gastroc raise exercise can cause the hamstring muscles to develop greater mass and strength. This exercise, therefore, can be of great value not only to athletes but also to bodybuilders interested in developing maximum muscle mass on the back side of the thigh. In addition, execution of this exercise helps to produce a better balance between the hamstring and quadriceps muscles. Equally important is the fact that the gluteus maximus is also maximally involved because in the starting position the hip is flexed a full 90 degrees (for those with sufficient hamstring flexibility).

- The glute-ham-gastroc raise exercise works the gastrocnemius muscle in an unusual manner. Instead of ankle joint flexion as used in the heel raise or the knee curl in which your lower leg moves toward your thigh, in this exercise your foot and lower leg remain stationary and your thigh moves toward your shin. Because your body is held rigid, in line with the thigh, it is more accurate to say that your entire body moves toward your lower leg during the knee joint flexion. In this movement there is much greater resistance and thus a stronger stimulus for additional development.

PART TWO

The Midsection

5 The Spine: The Abdominals

ANATOMY OF THE SPINE

The spinal column is a unique and well-designed structure. It has a total of 24 vertebrae, and because each vertebra must support the weight of all the body parts above it, the lower vertebrae are much larger than the upper ones. Attached to the thoracic (chest) vertebrae are 12 pairs of ribs which form the skeleton of the thorax (chest cavity).

Cartilaginous intervertebral discs are located between the vertebrae. The discs are composed of a jell-like mass surrounded by a heavy, strong layer of fibrocartilage. The discs permit motion between the vertebrae and also provide a cushion for them. The vertebrae are held together by muscles and ligaments which extend from the skull down to the sacrum.

The spine has four normal curves which can be seen when it is viewed from the side. The cervical (neck) and lumbar (lower back) curves are concave to the rear, and the thoracic (chest) and sacral (pelvic) curves are convex to the rear. There is a smooth transition from one curve into another. This arrangement gives effective support to the spine and allows for independent movement of different sections of the spine.

Movements of the spine take place by compression and deformation of the elastic intervertebral discs and by the gliding of the articular processes of the vertebrae (protusions at the top and bottom of each vertebra) upon one another.

The range of movement of each individual spinal (vertebral) joint is very small. However, when many vertebrae are involved at one time, the total movement of all the joints can appear to be very large. The limited range of interspinal motion is due to the tight ligaments and the shape and positioning of the interlocking parts of the vertebrae. In the thoracic area the ribs limit the range of motion.

BASIC MOVEMENTS OF THE SPINE

Four basic movements are possible in the spine:

1. Flexion, or forward bending of the spine, in which the anterior surfaces of the vertebrae move closer to one another.
2. Extension, or the return from a position of flexion to the anatomical position. Going beyond the anatomical position (bending backward) is called hyperextension. Keep in mind that slight hyperextension is the normal position of the lumbar spine (also known as slight lordosis).
3. Lateral flexion, or bending sideways to the right or left. In this action the shoulders move toward the hip, or the hips (pelvis) move toward the shoulders (when the hips are in a non-support or hanging support position). Lateral flexion and extension are discussed in Chapter 6.

4. Shoulder rotation, a twisting action around the long axis of the spinal column. In this movement the shoulders (shoulder girdle) are in motion. However, if you are positioned so that your lower body is hanging, supported by your upper body, you can use the same muscles to rotate your hips to the right or left when your shoulders remain stationary. This is known as transverse pelvic girdle rotation, which can also occur when you are standing, but in that case the action is in the hip joints, not the midsection.

MAJOR MUSCLES INVOLVED

The muscles that produce spinal movement exist in pairs, one on each side of the spine (and abdomen). They can function independently or together. The anterior spinal muscles do not attach directly to the vertebrae. This includes all the abdominal muscles. When the abdominals contract (shorten) and move the rib cage down and/or the pelvic girdle up, the spine is pulled into flexion.

Spinal flexion involves the abdominal muscles, which include the rectus abdominis and the internal and external obliques (see Figure 5.1). The rectus abdominis is a fairly slender muscle that runs vertically across the front of the abdominal wall. It originates on the crest of the pubis and inserts on the cartilage of the fifth, sixth, and seventh ribs. The right and left halves are separated by a tendinous strip about an inch wide called the linea alba. The muscle fibers run parallel to one another and are crossed by three tendons, which provide the divisions usually seen in a person with little fat in the abdominal area and a well-developed rectus abdominis muscle, commonly known as being "ripped." The rectus abdominis follows a curved line when at rest, and when contracted it becomes straight.

The external oblique, which covers the front sides of the abdomen, is located on both sides of the rectus abdominis. It is attached to the lower eight ribs at the upper end (origin) and the front half of the ilium, the crest of the pubis, and the linea alba at the lower end (insertion). The fibers run diagonally upward and sideward from the lower attachment on both sides of the abdomen and form a letter V when viewed from the front.

The internal oblique is located directly underneath the external oblique, and at its upper end its fibers run at nearly right angles to the external oblique fibers, forming an inverted letter V when viewed from the front. At the lower end, however, the internal oblique fibers are almost horizontal. The internal oblique muscle originates on the lumbar fascia, the anterior crest of the ilium, and the outer half of the inguinal ligament. At the upper end it inserts on the cartilage of the eighth, ninth, and tenth ribs and the linea alba. Both the internal and external oblique muscles cover a very wide area on the front side of the abdomen.

The internal and external oblique muscles are responsible for rotation of the upper and lower trunk, lateral flexion, and flexion of the spine. In rotation, when the shoulder girdle is held in place, contraction of these muscles will rotate the pelvic girdle. If the pelvic girdle is held stationary, rotation of the upper trunk (shoulders) occurs.

To produce this rotation, the externals on one side of the abdomen combine with the internals on the other side to create a diagonal pull across the abdomen. For example, the lower left side and the upper right side or the lower right side and the upper left side combine to form a long line of pull in the rotary actions.

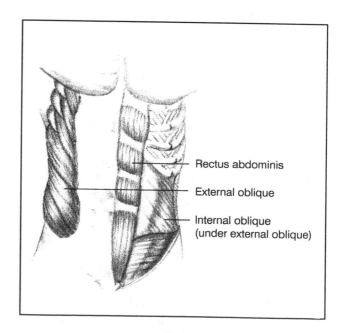

Rectus abdominis

External oblique

Internal oblique
(under external oblique)

Figure 5.1
Anterior view of the abdomen

Although it is not involved in movement of the spine, it is important to mention the deepest layer of abdominal muscles, which is called the transversus abdominis. Its origin is on the outer third of the inguinal ligament, the crest of the ilium, the cartilage of the lower six ribs, and the lumbar fascia. It inserts on the crest of the pubis and the iliopectineal line and the linea alba, where the muscles join in the middle. The transversus abdominis plays a very important role in holding the viscera in to produce a flat abdominal wall. In addition, this muscle plays an important role in forced expiration.

ABDOMINAL EXERCISES

■ Sit-Up (Curl-Up)

Many bodybuilders, athletes, and fitness buffs ignore the sit-up and do the crunch instead, which is like the sit-up except that you do not rise up as much. There is no questioning the fact that the crunch is an effective exercise, but the sit-up can also be as, or even more, effective. Thus, it should remain in your repertoire of abdominal exercises. However, if you have back problems or are predisposed to back problems, you should avoid doing the sit-up.

Major muscles and actions involved

The upper rectus abdominis and internal and external obliques are involved in spinal flexion (see Figure 5.2). This is not a separate group of muscles; rather, only the upper portion of the entire muscle is in action, as substantiated by EMG (electromyogram) studies. In this exercise your head and shoulders are lifted and rotated toward your hips.

Sports uses

The sit-up exercise is important for all athletes who throw implements with maximum force (baseball, football, javelin, shot) and for those who perform acrobatic-type movements such as diving, trampolining, and gymnastics. Upper abdominal development is very important to bodybuilders because these muscles show the ripped effect. Athletes who must handle heavy loads or stabilize their spines need strong abdominal muscles to maintain firm midsections.

Execution

Lie down on your back with your legs bent at the knees and your feet either free or secured. Keep your arms alongside your body, or fold them on your chest if you want more resistance (see Photo 5.1). When you are ready, inhale slightly more than usual and hold your breath as you raise your head and shoulders off the floor, concentrating on curling your upper trunk as much as possible. Rise up and over until your trunk is 30–45 degrees off the floor (see Photo 5.2). At this point begin to exhale and return to the initial position under control. Relax your muscles momentarily so that your head again rests on the floor and then repeat at a moderate rate of speed.

Comments

• There is considerable controversy over whether your legs should be straight or bent at the knees when you do the sit-up. In general, your knees should always be bent when your legs are held down or secured in some other way. When you attempt to do a sit-up with your legs straight, the psoas muscle (which is a hip joint flexor and is attached to the lower vertebrae) comes into play. This muscle can cause the lower spine to hyperextend (arch), which can cause lower back problems if the stress is sufficiently great. However, it is important to understand that the pull of the psoas on the spine is critical only when your body is in a straight-line position on the floor. Once you have a slight flexion of the spine, as you do in the beginning positions of the sit-up and crunch exercises, and you can hold that position, it is impossible for the psoas to hyperextend the spine. Flattening the lumbar area of the spine by contracting your abdominals and tilting your pelvis backwards as you begin to do the straight-leg sit-up will remove the possibility of hyperextension, and therefore, performing sit-ups in this manner is not dangerous. If it were, many other exercises would be dangerous as well, including the hanging leg raise; the knee-up and other exercises which involve hip flexion before spinal flexion; running, especially sprinting; and even walking fast when the hip flexors are used greatly.
• The sit-up has also been negatively criticized because the hip flexors are also involved when your legs are secured. However, there is noth-

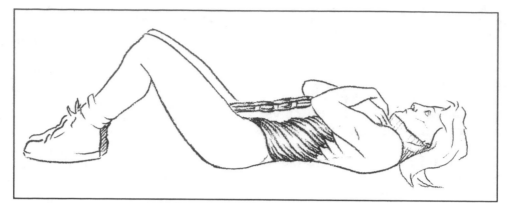

Figure 5.2
Muscles used in the sit-up

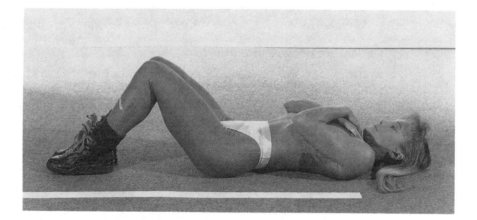

Photo 5.1

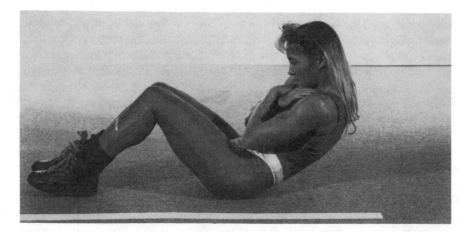

Photo 5.2

ing wrong with hip flexor involvement. In fact, it is beneficial to develop these muscles in order to keep your pelvis properly aligned. Thus, by doing a sit-up with your knees bent and your feet secured, you get development not only of the upper abdominals but of the hip flexors as well. In essence, you work the mutual relationship between these muscles.

- In addition, the full sit-up (to an erect sitting position) has been criticized as being detrimental to the lower spine, but in fact it is only detrimental if you maintain the curled-up position past 30–45 degrees above the floor. You should not rise up higher than 45 degrees above the floor, because when you do, the vertebrae are opened excessively on the posterior side, which causes severe squeezing of the anterior discs. However, if you straighten your spine as you pass the 45-degree mark (as most people do naturally), it is perfectly safe to continue the movement to 90 degrees—but not beyond. Doing so will again place excessive strain on your spine.

- Often the terms "stomach muscles" and "tummy muscles" are used to describe the abdominal muscles. This is grossly incorrect. The stomach muscle is a smooth muscle which contracts the walls of the stomach as an aid to digesting food. The abdominal muscles, however, are skeletal muscles which are responsible for moving body parts. Thus, the two terms should not be interchanged.

- The sit-up exercise should be modified gradually as your muscles develop in order to increase the resistance or to make the exercise more difficult. The amount of modification will, of course, depend upon your objectives. Advanced sit-ups, including the basic sit-up, can be quite stressful and should be done only in relation to your level of preparation and ability. Sit-ups may cause pain and injury to people who have weak abdominal muscles, and it may be safer for those people to do crunches instead.

To increase the difficulty of the sit-up, use the slant (incline) board and gradually increase its slope, or hold weights on your chest as you do the exercise. A combination of both will increase the difficulty even more. However, do not make the board too steep because this can greatly increase the blood pressure in your head as you do the exercise.

- Some fitness authorities believe that you should exhale on the exertion when you do the sit-up or crunch. Their reasoning is that when you hold your breath, your abdominals will protrude as you do the sit-up and thus you will have a protruding abdominal wall as a result. To counteract this, they recommend that you exhale forcefully to suck in your abdominals as you do the sit-up so that your muscles will develop inwardly rather than outwardly.

In theory, this sounds very effective. However, from a physiological and anatomical standpoint, this can be a very dangerous practice. When you exhale before and during the rising-up portion of the sit-up, you do not have enough intra-abdominal pressure to stabilize your spine. In essence, your spine will be very weak during the exercise, which can place undue pressure on the intervertebral discs. Also, when you hold your breath during the exertion, not only are you much stronger (up to 20 percent), but you allow the rectus abdominis and the obliques to shorten maximally, which is very important for developing strength. Keep in mind that the greater the strength of these muscles, the more effective they will be in holding in the internal organs and creating a flat abdominal wall. (However, it should be noted that the rotational exercises, and not the sit-up, are the key exercises for developing a flat abdominal wall.)

When you do sit-ups or crunches, the abdominal muscles expand as they shorten. This is how it should be. Don't all the other muscles in the body expand when contracted? Of course they do, and so it is with the abdominals in the sit-up. However, the abdominal muscles are also being shortened. When you suck in your abdominals, they must contract in a curved shape, which is very ineffective. It is analogous to placing a tight strap around the biceps muscle when it is relaxed and then trying to contract the muscle. It doesn't work!

It should also be mentioned that holding your breath during the exertion is a natural phenomenon, especially when the exercise becomes difficult. It is your body's way of trying to create greater force and maintaining a safe position.

- To develop more of the oblique muscles, many individuals do the sit-up or crunch with a twist. However, these exercises are dangerous and you should not do them. The reason is that when you do a sit-up, your spine is flexed, and if you then twist, great shearing forces are created on the anterior aspects of the vertebrae. Therefore, you should do rotation only when your spine is in its normal anatomical position. If you wish to involve some of the rotational muscles, you can lie on the floor and do a single-shoulder lift. However, this exercise involves mainly the upper portion of the abdominals and not all of the rotator muscles.

• Many people now do the crunch exercise because it does not involve the hip flexors. The crunch is a good exercise, especially for those who feel pain or discomfort when they do sit-ups. The crunch also involves the upper abdominal muscles, but it does not ensure a maximum range of motion. When your feet are not secured, you do not have a firm base against which to work to get maximum abdominal contractions.

• The crunch is done just like the sit-up except that you raise your head and shoulders only about 15–20 degrees off the floor. However, when you do the crunch, your abdominals contract strongly and shorten to 30 or even 45 degrees, depending upon your flexibility in the waist. Because of this, the sit-up is preferred for more complete shortening of the abdominals and for greater strength.

You can also perform the crunch with your legs up in the air, but if you do the exercise like this, you must automatically contract your lower abdominals to stabilize your pelvis so your hip muscles can stabilize your legs. When your legs rest on a bench, your pelvis is not stabilized, which creates slack in the upper rectus abdominis. Thus, when you do the crunch, you do not feel your muscles truly shortening until you are at the uppermost position. This defeats one of the main reasons for performing the exercise, but it also explains why many individuals do crunches over a very short range of motion.

When you do the crunch, it is important that you return to the initial position, where your head is in contact with the floor, because this allows your muscles to stretch back to their original shape. Too often people do not return to the initial position when they do the crunch,

and, consequently, their muscles shorten, which results in a pulling of the rib cage downward and poor posture (a forward chest and head).

■ Abdominal Machine Crunch

Also very effective for upper abdominal development are exercises done on exercise machines such as the one made by Keiser. These machines are effective in duplicating the crunch movement and in stabilizing the spine for a limited range of motion. Thus, abdominal machines make a good variant to your abdominal work and should be a part of your arsenal of exercises.

Major muscles and actions involved

The upper rectus abdominis and the internal and external obliques are involved (see Figure 5.3). These muscles are responsible for flexion of the spine with the upper trunk curling toward the hips. After the crunch action the movement continues via hip joint flexion, during which the abdominal muscles undergo isometric contraction to hold the bent-over position.

Sports uses

The sports uses are the same as for the sit-up. However, when using a machine, you get the added benefit of the isometric contraction through a good portion of the total range of motion.

Execution

Execution on the Keiser machine will be described, but it is basically the same as on other machines. Adjust the seat so that when you are properly positioned the chest pad is on your upper chest. Sit down and line your hips up with the axis of rotation of the machine. Grasp the handles in front of your chest and adjust the resistance (see Photo 5.3). When you are ready, inhale and hold your breath as you crunch forward and move your trunk approximately 60 degrees forward (see Photo 5.4). Then exhale and return to the starting position and repeat.

Comments

• For variety, this exercise can also be done with your hands behind your back or behind your neck. However, the behind-the-neck position is not recommended because doing the exercise in this manner can strain the neck.

- As you do the repetitions, you can change the resistance during the movement either on the crunching action phase or on the return. In this way you can gain greater eccentric or concentric strength at any point in the range of motion.

- The Keiser abdominal machine is effective for doing the crunch and holding this position. In so doing, you develop greater stabilizing strength of the spine, which is very important in many different exercises. In many activities this stabilization is needed when your trunk is erect, so to develop further stabilizing strength you can also increase the resistance when your body is upright and then do an isometric contraction in the erect position. You will notice that you will feel the tension in your abdominals as well as your hip flexors, and this is an indication that abdominal machine exercises are effective in working the relationship between the spinal and hip flexors.

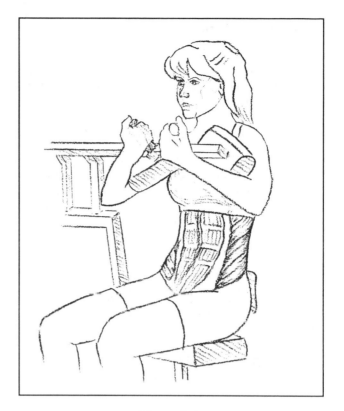

Figure 5.3
Muscles used in the abdominal machine crunch

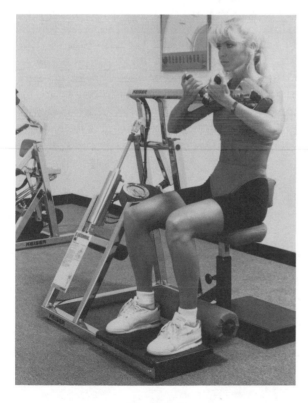

Photo 5.3

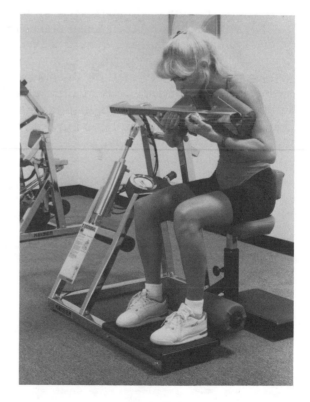

Photo 5.4

■ Reverse Sit-Up

Crunches and sit-ups develop only the upper abdominals. To develop the lower abdominals, you must do the reverse sit-up.

Major muscles and actions involved

In this exercise the lower portion of the abdominal muscles (especially the rectus abdominis) performs spinal flexion (see Figure 5.4). In this action the pelvic girdle rotates up and toward the upper trunk. This is the opposite of what occurs in the sit-up or crunch.

Sports uses

The reverse sit-up is an important exercise for all sports that require abdominal strength to rotate the pelvis posteriorly to produce a maximum range of motion to lift the legs up high. Thus, gymnasts should perform this exercise to develop the muscles needed to raise their legs to a 90-degree angle or higher in many of the stunts executed on the apparatus and in free exercise. Likewise, it is an important exercise for dancers, especially for developing the muscles needed to raise the legs in ballet leaps and in modern dance. Runners should do the reverse sit-up so that they are able to raise their knees sufficiently for maximum stride length, whereas kickers in soccer, football, karate, and rugby should do the exercise to help them bring their thigh forward to execute powerful kicks. This exercise is especially important for women to eliminate the little "pouch" in the lower abdomen and to develop a relatively flat lower abdominal wall.

Execution

Lie on your back on an exercise mat or carpeted floor. Keep your arms alongside your body with your palms down and raise your thighs with your knees until your upper legs are vertical. This is the starting position (see Photo 5.5).

When you are ready, inhale slightly more than usual and then hold your breath as you raise your pelvis up and toward your shoulders until your hips are off the floor. Keep your knees bent tightly as you do this so the action is isolated to the lower abdominals. Push down with your hands to help raise your hips (and legs) and to ensure adequate rotation of the pelvic girdle. In the ending position your knees should be close to your chest (see Photo 5.6). Keep your head and shoulders as relaxed as possible throughout the upward movement. Exhale as you return to the initial position, stop, and then repeat.

Comments

- If you want to involve the upper abdominal muscles also, continue bringing your pelvis and bent legs up and over until your knees are above your head. Doing this produces a maximal stretch of the spine. However, this is an advanced movement and is not a key element of the reverse sit-up. The main factor in successful development is to have the pelvic girdle fully rotated off the floor, at which point the lower abdominal muscle fibers are maximally contracted. Also, going beyond this range can be detrimental for some individuals.

- In the beginning movement of this exercise, you may find it helpful to press hard with your hands against the floor to assist you in getting

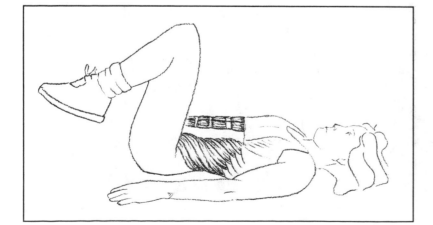

Figure 5.4
Muscles used in the reverse sit-up

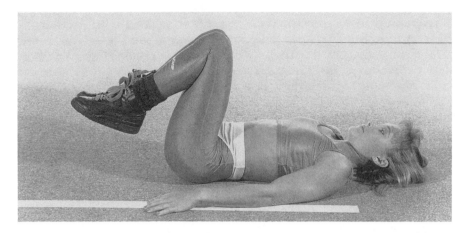

Photo 5.5

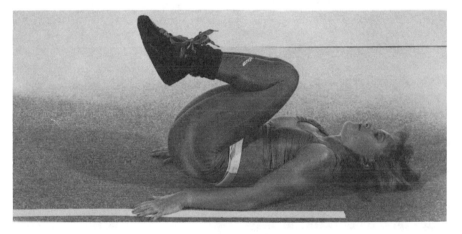

Photo 5.6

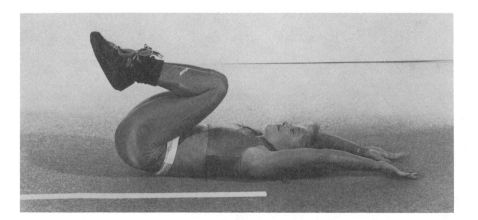

Photo 5.7

your pelvic girdle rotated up and over. But you should not do this continually as it may irritate your shoulders. More importantly, if you want maximum muscle involvement, you must use your lower abdominal muscles to start the pelvic girdle rotation. Thus, once you can do the exercise easily, you should place your arms over (or under) your head (see Photo 5.7). In this position you will have to rely solely on pulling with your lower abdominal muscles.

- Do not return your feet to the floor during execution because doing so creates momentum in your legs, which makes it easier for you to rotate your lower pelvis upward, which in turn means that the following initial stage of raising your legs is done, by your hip joint flexors, not your abdominals.

- As you become more proficient, to make the exercise even more difficult, do not return your thighs to the vertical position. Keep them bent toward your chest so that there is zero moving inertia and a maximum initial muscular contraction.

- To execute a more difficult version of the reverse sit-up, you can do the exercise on a slant board. In this case, you must hold onto something, which will automatically assist you in raising your pelvis. Execution is the same as on the floor.

- The reverse sit-up is an excellent stretching and strengthening exercise. When you bring your knees up close to your chest when your pelvic girdle rotates off the floor, you actually stretch your lower back muscles greatly. This is not a passive stretch but an active one because your abdominal muscles must contract strongly to place you in this position. Thus, you strengthen your abdominals as you stretch your lower back.

◼ Hanging Leg Raise

If you do not counteract the effects of weight training on your spine by doing flexibility exercises, in time you could develop spinal problems. To prevent this and to get great abdominal development at the same time, you should perform the hanging leg raise.

Major muscles and actions involved

Hanging and forearm-supported hanging leg raises involve the iliopsoas, the rectus femoris,

and the pectineus in hip flexion and the rectus abdominis and external oblique muscles in spinal flexion (see Figure 5.5). In this action you raise your legs, either held straight or bent, toward your trunk from the vertical position. When your legs get past 45–60 degrees of upward motion, your pelvic girdle begins to rotate posteriorly, that is, your iliac crests move backward and your pelvis moves forward and upward to assist in continuing to raise your legs.

Sports uses

Hip and spinal flexion and the muscles involved are needed in all actions which require raising your legs high in front of your body. Thus, the sports uses are the same as for the reverse sit-up.

Development of the muscles involved is also important for proper spinal posture in various movements because these muscles stabilize the pelvic girdle (together with the erector spinae and the hip extensors).

For bodybuilders, doing this exercise through a maximum range of motion is very important

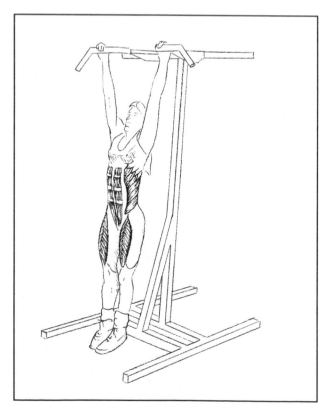

Figure 5.5
Muscles used in the hanging leg raise

for achieving the ripped effect. Everyone also benefits from the spinal stretching to maintain spinal flexibility. Hanging is very important in keeping the vertebrae apart to prevent pinching of the nerves.

Execution

Execution of the hanging leg raise is basically the same as execution of the support leg raise done on the hip flexor apparatus. Therefore, the two exercises will be described simultaneously.

Variant 1—*Support leg raise (knee-up):* Grasp a high bar or hip flexor apparatus with your forearms supported on the bar and your body hanging vertically. When you are in position, inhale and hold your breath as you bend and raise your knees until your thighs are horizontal or higher. Exhale and return your legs to the vertical position under control. Relax for a moment and then repeat. Execute the up phase at a moderate rate of speed.

Variant 2—*Hanging leg raise:* This is a more difficult exercise. Grasp a high bar with your hands so that your entire body can hang vertically, using a pronated grip to prevent swinging (see Photo 5.8). When you are ready, inhale slightly more than usual and hold your breath as you raise your legs in hip flexion, keeping them straight (or slightly bent). Raise your legs until they are horizontal (so your body forms an L) or higher (see Photo 5.9). Exhale as you return to the starting position under control. Relax for a moment and then repeat. Execute at a moderate rate of speed.

Comments

- As a general rule, weights are not needed in this exercise, especially if you keep your legs straight and if you raise them sufficiently high. The weight and long length of the legs provide great resistance. However, if you want more resistance, you can wear ankle weights.
- Hanging leg raises are maximally effective for development of your lower and upper abdominals if your legs are raised to a maximally high position (maximum posterior pelvic girdle rotation), as when you touch your toes to your hands. This range is not possible in the forearm support variant, but in that variant you can still raise your feet above the horizontal.

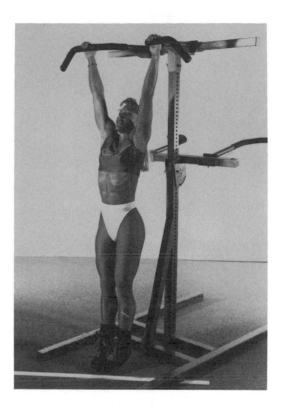

Photo 5.8

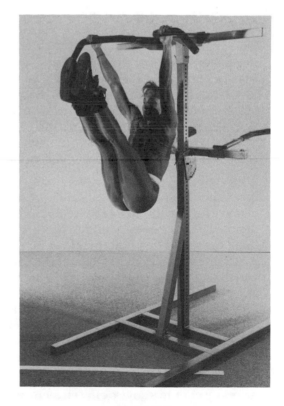

Photo 5.9

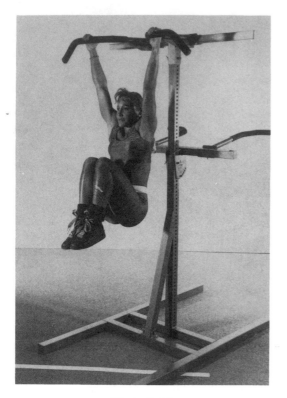

Photo 5.10

When executing maximum range movements, the hip flexor muscles remain under isometric contraction to hold your legs in the hip-flexed position when your abdominals go into action to rotate your pelvis. Also, when your hip flexor muscles are in action, your abdominals remain in isometric contraction to stabilize and hold the pelvic girdle stationary. This is needed to allow the hip flexors a base upon which they can pull the legs up.

• If lifting your legs and keeping them straight is too difficult, you should begin doing this exercise with your knees bent (see Photo 5.10). By bending your knees, you cut down the resistance by about one-half. In addition, this automatically relaxes your hamstring muscles, which, in turn, allows you to go through a fuller range of motion in hip flexion. When the bent-leg knee-ups are easy to do, gradually straighten your legs to make the exercise more difficult. Work up to the point where you can keep your legs straight throughout the entire range of motion.

• As many people know, doing straight-leg raises while you are lying on your back may be in-

jurious to the spine if the pelvic girdle is not held stable by the abdominals. In the support straight-leg raises, however, the abdominals automatically undergo contraction at the very beginning of the movement. Because of this, the hanging leg raise is a safe exercise for development of the hip flexors together with the abdominal muscles.

■ Reverse Trunk Twist

Sit-ups, reverse sit-ups, hanging leg raises, and other abdominal exercises that involve spinal flexion do not produce a full contraction from the internal and external obliques and therefore these muscles do not get maximum development. The reverse trunk twist can be performed to obtain maximum development of these muscles.

Major muscles and actions involved

In the reverse trunk twist, the internal and external oblique (abdominal) muscles are involved in rotation of the pelvic girdle (see Figure 5.6). In this action your shoulders remain in place while your pelvis (and legs) rotates to the left and right with the axis in the trunk.

Sports uses

The action of pelvic girdle rotation and the muscles involved are critical in all throwing, hitting, punching, and kicking actions. For example, when you throw a baseball or football, the oblique muscles pull your shoulders around. The same thing happens when you hit the ball in baseball and softball and when you execute different shots in sports such as tennis and racquetball. The muscles used in the reverse trunk twist are also involved in rotating your upper trunk in various punches used in boxing and karate.

Rotation of the pelvic girdle is also needed in various side approach soccer kicks and in kicking in football (especially field goals). When you run, the obliques help to hold your pelvis in place so that it does not rotate with each forward leg action. When you lift weights, these muscles and actions are very important for holding your midsection firmly and to prevent rotation or bending of the spine, as, for example, when you do the overhead press. In bodybuilding this

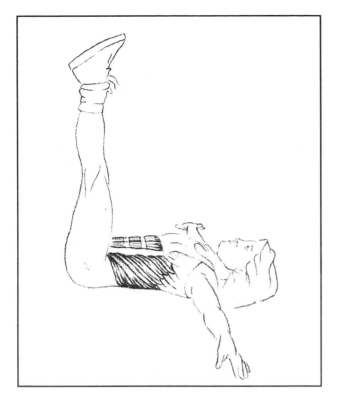

Figure 5.6
Muscles used in the reverse trunk twist

exercise is very important for development of the muscles on the front sides of the abdominal wall.

Execution

Lie face up on the floor with your arms out to the sides and your palms down. Your arms should be perpendicular to your trunk so that your body forms a letter T. Keeping your legs straight and your feet together, raise your legs to a 90-degree angle to the floor. (If you have tight hamstrings, bend your knees slightly to reduce the tension.) Keep your feet together and maintain this leg-trunk position throughout the entire exercise (see Photo 5.11).

When you are ready, lower your legs to one side while continuing to hold the 90-degree angle in your hip joints. Touch the floor with the outside of your lower foot, keeping your shoulders and arms in full contact with the floor (see Photo 5.12). Then inhale and raise your legs back to the initial position and, without stopping, over to the opposite side until your feet touch, again keeping your shoulders in contact with the floor. Exhale as you lower your legs and then repeat, alternating sides.

Comments

• If you find this exercise difficult in the early stages, bend your knees fully so that your thighs are lowered to the sides (see Photo 5.13 and Photo 5.14). The greater the knee bend, the "shorter" the legs and the easier it is to execute the exercise. The straighter the legs, the more difficult the exercise. When doing the exercise with your legs held straight becomes easy, you can add weights to your feet to increase the resistance.

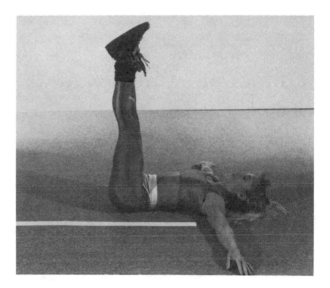

Photo 5.11

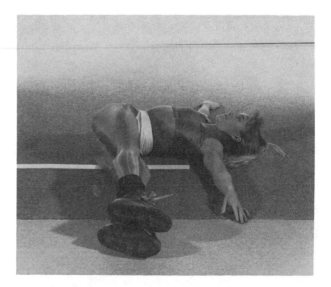

Photo 5.12

- If your shoulders come off the floor as your legs are lowered to the side, have someone hold them down. With increased flexibility, you should be able to do the exercise by yourself.
- The diagonal muscle fibers of the internal and external oblique muscles form a strong, interlacing network, which, when shortened or well developed, forms a relatively flat sheet that produces the flat abdominal wall. Keep in mind that the rectus abdominis is a curved muscle in its natural state and only straightens when it is under contraction. This can be

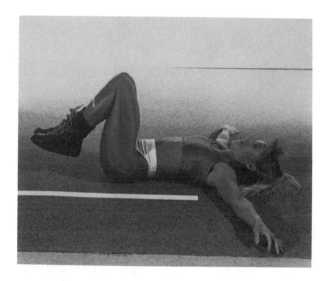

Photo 5.13

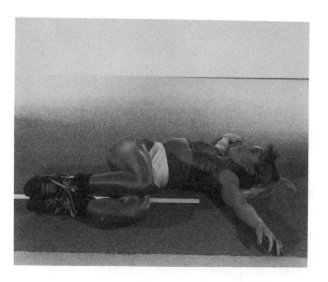

Photo 5.14

illustrated by recalling the days when women wore corsets. When the corset was laced up, the strings were pulled in from the sides to flatten the front. It was not tightened from top to bottom as the muscles are when you do sit-ups, crunches, and reverse sit-ups.

- Another muscle which plays an important role in maintaining a flat abdominal wall is the transversus abdominis. Because of its structure and deep location, it is ideally suited to keep the abdominal wall flat and not allow it to protrude. However, the only time the transversus contracts strongly is in forced expiration, which also involves the other abdominal muscles. The transversus abdominis is not involved in any movements of the spine as are the other abdominal muscles. Therefore, to develop the transversus (as well as the other abdominal muscles), it is necessary to do breathing exercises, especially those that involve full and forceful exhalation.

  One of the best resistive breathing devices to use for forced expiration is the Sports Breather. In essence, the Sports Breather is a small device with a mouthpiece and adjustable openings for air to enter and exit. With this device you can increase the resistance in both inhalation and exhalation, which forces the muscles to work harder. Preliminary studies have demonstrated the great effectiveness of this device in increasing chest size and in decreasing waist size. In addition, the Sports Breather helps to improve sports performances, especially in those sports that require endurance.

- The reverse trunk twist is also a very good exercise for developing midsection flexibility together with strength. This occurs when you can do the exercise without having anyone holding you and with your shoulders and arms in full contact with the floor. (It should also be noted that the latissimus dorsi is also stretched during execution.) Flexibility coupled with strength is a major deterrent to injuries of the spine. Thus, the reverse trunk twist can be considered a key exercise in the development of a healthy lower back.

- Another benefit of doing the reverse trunk twist is that it produces moderate development of the spinal muscles (the muscles that hold the vertebrae together and twist the spine). However, for true development of these muscles to prevent many typical back problems, you should do back raises and back raises with a twist.

■ Twisting

When you do the reverse trunk twist, your hips and legs are in motion. The reverse action, twisting, is done by keeping your hips stabilized and putting your shoulders into motion. This is a great warm-up activity that develops flexibility and some strength in the waist. However, as simple as twisting may appear, it can be dangerous if done incorrectly.

Major muscles and actions involved

Spinal rotation, in which your shoulders rotate around your spine, occurs in twisting. To produce this rotation, the externals on one side of your abdomen combine with the internals on the other side, so that there is a diagonal pull across the abdomen when you turn in each direction (see Figure 5.7). Also involved to some extent are the erector spinae muscles on the spine. Depending upon your flexibility, there may also be some transverse pelvic girdle rotation which involves the medial and lateral rotator muscles of the hip joints.

Sports uses

These are the same as for the reverse trunk twist. The twisting exercise is used mainly for warm-up and for increasing your range of motion, but if the repetitions are sufficiently high, you can also gain some muscular development.

Execution

Stand with your feet wider than shoulder-width apart, and place a Dyna-Flex Pole or similar pole across your shoulders. Grasp the bar with your arms at the ends of the bar. Keep your spine in its normal anatomical slightly arched position and bend your knees slightly (see Photo 5.15).

When you are ready, hold your body firmly and rotate it at a moderate rate of speed to one side as far as you can go until the bar is pointing to the front and back (see Photo 5.16). Then reverse directions and repeat the movement, alternating sides for the duration of the exercise. For proper and safe execution of this exercise, it is important that you make no quick or jerky actions in the movement. To assist in doing this, you should isometrically contract your leg and hip muscles to hold your body in place as you rotate. The rotation should be limited to your shoulders.

Comments

- You should not move too quickly when rotating your shoulders. If you do, a lot of momentum may develop, which makes it difficult to stop and reverse the twist in the end position. Keep in mind that very quick changes in direction can injure your spine.
- The key to effective execution of this exercise is to go through a full range of motion (approximately 180 degrees, 90 degrees on each side). Your pelvis should be held in place and when necessary rotated slightly to act as a safety valve to take some of the strain off your back in stopping and changing directions. When your pelvic girdle rotates, the action is in your hip joints (medial and lateral position), and this action tends to act as a shock absorber. You should never twist so much that the rotation goes into your knees because doing so causes great shearing forces that can injure the knees. This is why you should always keep your knees bent as you execute this exercise.

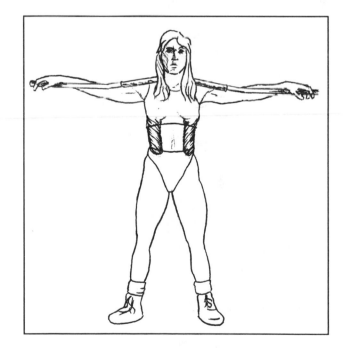

Figure 5.7
Muscles used in twisting

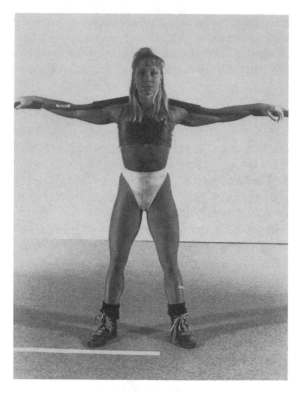

Photo 5.15

- For greater isolation of the midsection rotator muscles, you can do this exercise sitting down, which will eliminate involvement of the hip and knee joints. You may also find that the range of motion decreases somewhat when you do this exercise sitting down. To ensure a stable position, you should press with your thighs against the bench as you change directions.
- Twisting while standing up is not as effective for strength development as twisting while lying down. The reason for this is that when you are standing, you do not work against gravity. Shoulder girdle rotations done from a horizontal position, as, for example the Russian twist or the reverse trunk twist, are much more effective.
- When you are twisting at a fairly vigorous pace, the rotational muscles of your trunk develop some muscle resiliency from the reversals of direction. However, be sure not to go too fast. To allow for greater effectiveness and safety in switching directions quickly, you can use weighted balls such as D-Balls, whose firmness for gripping can be regulated.

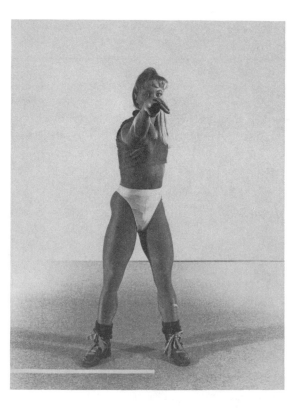

Photo 5.16

■ Glute-Ham Developer Sit-Up

Many people do sit-ups or crunches to develop their abdominals, but these exercises have limited effectiveness. However, because of the great intensity and levels of performance needed for almost all sports, athletes and bodybuilders should do exercises commensurate with their levels of ability—exercises which produce a greater development of the midsection that is needed for lifting heavy weights or executing skills that require great force or speed. Doing Glute-Ham Developer (GHD) sit-ups will give you the greater intensity needed for the highest levels of athletic performance.

Major muscles and actions involved

In the GHD sit-up the abdominal muscles are responsible for spinal flexion (see Figures 5.8 and 5.9). In this action your abdominal muscles pull your head and shoulders up and forward from a slightly lower than horizontal position. In some variants the hip flexors contract to rotate the pelvis (together with the trunk) up and forward from a slightly below horizontal position on an axis in the hip joint.

Sports uses

The GHD sit-up is an important exercise for all sports that require firm stabilization of the spine, especially for sports such as football and rugby in which great forces applied to the upper body must be withstood. The stabilization is also needed for many sports movements, especially when objects are lifted overhead or when force is applied from the legs to the arms as in the tennis serve.

The variant which also involves the hip joint is an important exercise to do if you engage in sports which require you to lift your legs high when you are in a hanging or horizontal position. This action is needed by gymnasts in a multitude of movements on the apparatus and in free exercise. In addition, it is needed by modern dancers and ballet dancers when they leap high, trampolinists, divers, acrobats (who hold an L position), and so on. These exercises are also very important for baseball pitchers and football quarterbacks.

The muscles and actions involved in GHD sit-ups are very important for pulling the trunk forward to create more force and speed when throwing. Thus, the exercise is valuable for javelin throwers, tennis players in serving, soccer players in kicking and in the throw-in, and volleyball players in spiking. Swimmers, especially in the freestyle and butterfly, must also have very strong lower abdominals and hip flex-

ors to maintain proper body position and for force in kicking.

The GHD sit-up is very effective as an advanced exercise for producing a flat and well-defined abdominal wall. Because of this, the exercise is very important to bodybuilders and fitness buffs. In addition, a strong abdominal wall together with strong erector spinae muscles of the lower back are the keys to injury prevention and a pain-free back.

Execution

Variant 1—*Upper abdominals:* Adjust the BFS Glute-Ham Developer so that when you sit on the seat with your feet secured between the rollers and against the back plate, your pelvis will be in full support on the seat. Your legs should be straight and horizontal and your trunk vertical. Place your hands on your chest. Inhale a bit more than usual and then hold your breath as you slowly lower your trunk until it is slightly below the level of the horizontal. In this position your head and shoulders will be below the level of your hips (see Photo 5.17).

After reaching the bottom position, keep holding your breath and slowly curl back up to about a 45-degree angle and then straighten your back as you return to the upright position and exhale (see Photo 5.18). As a general rule, in the bottom position you should have a slight arch in your lumbar spine, and in the upright position your

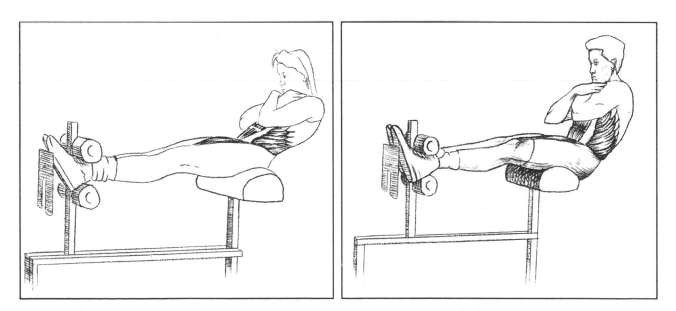

Figure 5.8
Muscles used in the GHD sit-up, variant 1

Figure 5.9
Muscles used in the GHD sit-up, variant 2

back should be slightly flexed. Do each repetition at a slow to moderate rate of speed. Initially, you will not need weights, but when you become proficient at this exercise and wish to increase the difficulty, hold a barbell plate on your chest with both your hands.

Variant 2—*Lower abdominals:* Adjust the BFS GHD so that when you are seated, support will be under the back side of your upper thighs. Your feet should be secured between the rollers, and your legs should be fully extended. Inhale slightly more than usual and hold your breath as you lower your body back and down until your trunk is below the level of your thighs (see Photo 5.19). Your legs should remain straight at all times. When you are in the correct position, you will feel tension in your abdominal, hip, and thigh muscles. Curl your trunk up about 30

degrees and then use your hip flexors to return to the upright position and exhale. At this time your spine should be slightly rounded (see Photo 5.20). Do each repetition at a slow to moderate rate of speed. To increase the resistance, hold weights on your chest.

Comments

• It is important to do the movements in this exercise at a slow to moderate speed and under control at all times. You should not make any quick or jerky movements because these can prove dangerous to your spine or hips. When you move slowly to the down position, concentrate on a slight arch in the lower back and a stretching of your abdominal muscles. Feel your abdominal muscles contracting as you rise up.

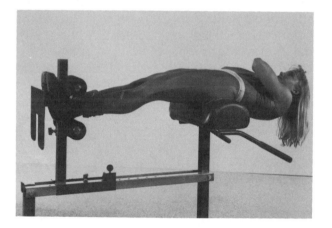

Photo 5.17

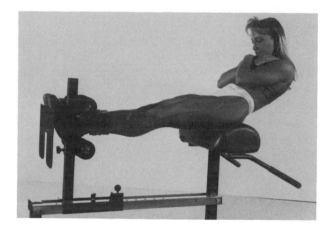

Photo 5.18

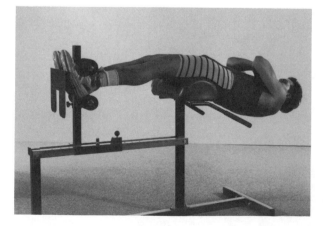

Photo 5.19

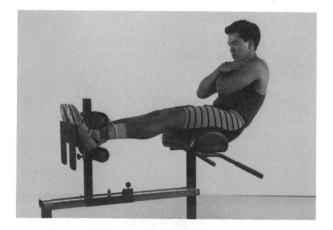

Photo 5.20

• The hip flexors are involved in both variants. However, it is important to understand that throughout this entire exercise, your abdominals are under very strong contraction. They, in essence, hold your spine in place and do not allow your hip flexors to hyperextend your spine. Because of this, the GHD sit-up is a very safe but advanced exercise. It should also be noted that the hip flexors and abdominals are under constant contraction supporting the trunk in this non-support position (when the trunk is beyond the hips). When you lean back, your muscles undergo a strong eccentric contraction (which is also responsible for muscle development) and then a concentric-isometric contraction on the way up. Thus, the muscles undergo all three muscle contraction regimes.

• If you keep your legs straight, it is very difficult (if not impossible) to lower your trunk so that your head is pointing vertically toward the floor with your back excessively hyperextended. If this happens, you are in a potentially very dangerous position. Hanging down backwards as far as possible creates tremendous pressure on the posterior aspects of the discs, which is a leading cause of back problems. The key to successful execution of this exercise is to lower your trunk so that there is approximately 15–20 (30 maximum) degrees of hyperextension when doing the exercise. This is more than sufficient to produce a great training effect in the abdominals. If you drop lower, you are most likely bending your knees.

• The GHD sit-up is an advanced exercise and should not be undertaken by anyone who has a weak back. The forces involved in this exercise are great, and therefore your muscles should be well developed in order to do the exercise correctly and to create sufficient muscular force to hold your spine in a stable position at all times.

• As you start using weights, you will notice that the greater the amount of weight you use, the less is the flexion and hyperextension of the spine. The reason for this is that your muscles contract so tightly to hold your back in place that it is difficult for them to relax to produce sufficient arching and flexing of the spine. Thus, it is not always necessary to use excessive weights when doing this exercise. A slightly greater range of motion is often more desirable than merely holding your spine in place throughout the entire movement. In the latter case, the action is performed more by the hip flexors while the abdominals are under very strong isometric contraction. However, this is still effective for spinal stabilization.

• Variant 2, in which your hips are positioned beyond the seat, is especially effective for stressing the lower abdominals along with the hip flexors. This is a very good example of how the hip flexors and lower abdominals work in coordination when doing flexion of the trunk. Because they work together, this variant is especially important for athletes who must run and kick and who must raise their legs or trunks.

• An effective substitute for the GHD sit-up is the bench sit-up. To execute this exercise, sit on a bench and have someone (or something) hold your legs in place. A key safety factor in this version is maintaining yourself in a proper and stable position. Execution is the same as on the GHD.

■ Russian Twist

One of the key elements in many sports that require swinging a bat, racquet, or club, or throwing an implement such as a baseball, football, javelin, shot put, or discus, is a strong rotation of the trunk. In some cases the trunk rotation develops up to 50 percent of the total force generated. One of the best advanced exercises to develop rotational ability is the Russian twist.

Major muscles and actions involved

In this exercise there is shoulder girdle rotation, which involves the internal and external obliques (see Figure 5.10). In this action you rotate your shoulders a full 180 degrees from a starting horizontal position. The rectus abdominis and the erector spinae isometrically contract to hold your trunk level in the horizontal position.

Sports uses

The same as for the reverse trunk twist.

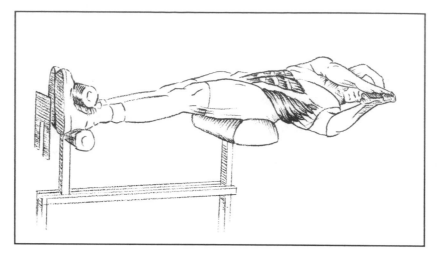

Figure 5.10
Muscles used in the Russian twist

Execution

To do this exercise without assistance, you should use a BFS Glute-Ham Developer. This is the only machine that has the adjustability needed to fit both short and tall individuals. Slide the foot placement unit so that when you sit with your pelvic girdle directly on top of the seat, your legs will be straight when your feet are secured. Lower your trunk to the horizontal position so that your entire body is parallel to the floor. Raise your arms so that they are perpendicular to your trunk, and hold a weight in your hands for greater resistance (see Photo 5.21). Hold your breath when you are in a horizontal position to make your midsection more rigid.

When you are ready, rotate your shoulders and arms as a unit to one side until your arms are relatively parallel to the floor and your shoulders are perpendicular to the floor (see Photo 5.22). Rotate back to the initial position and, without stopping, continue over to the other side until your arms are once again parallel to the floor and your shoulders are perpendicular to the floor. Continue this movement until you have completed the desired number of repetitions.

Breathing is very important in this exercise and must be adjusted to the way you perform the exercise. Most individuals should use the following pattern: As you rotate your shoulders to one side, quickly exhale near the bottom position, then inhale quickly, and then hold your breath as you rotate your shoulder-arm unit upward.

Repeat on the opposite side. The key is to breathe quickly so that you have maximum trunk stability.

Comments

- In this exercise you must hold your body level at all times. If you find yourself weakening and your back going into hyperextension or greater flexion, then immediately stop doing the exercise. Keep in mind that when you rotate with your spine in a flexed or hyperextended position, there are great shearing forces that could cause injury to the spine.
- The Russian twist is considered a specialized exercise because it closely duplicates some of the major skills involved in sports. For example, it duplicates the exact action of bringing the shoulders around in baseball hitting and pitching. It is one of the key actions in football quarterback throwing, and in the trunk rotation in forehand hits in the racquet sports, the golf swing, the shot put, and the discus.
- The Russian twist totally involves the abdominal muscles. The rectus abdominis remains under isometric contraction to hold the position while the internal and external obliques are involved in their major action of trunk rotation. In addition, because of the quick movement and somewhat forced inhalation and exhalation, there is strong contraction of the transversus abdominis, whose only function is forced expiration.

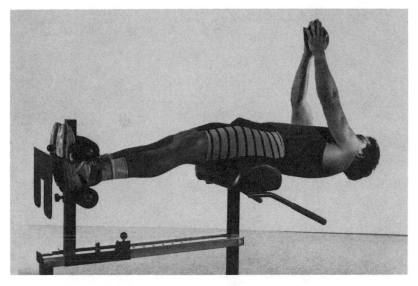

Photo 5.21

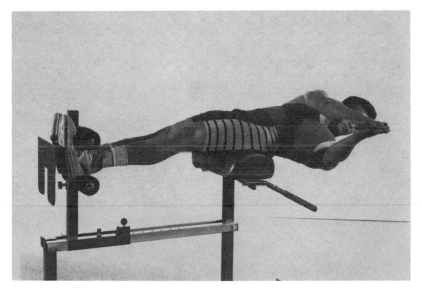

Photo 5.22

6 The Spine: Lower Back Muscles

There are many exercises used for development of the abdominal musculature but very few for the erector spinae. This is due partly to the phobia that existed about back extension exercises. Today, however, almost everyone is in agreement that extension exercises are very important for the development of a strong back. The best dynamic exercises are the back raise, the back raise with a twist, and the reverse back raise. To develop stabilization strength, you can use a back machine and perform other exercises.

MAJOR MUSCLES INVOLVED

Two sets of muscles are involved in extension of the spine: a deep spinal group and a superficial spinal group (see Figure 6.1).

The superficial group is collectively known as the erector spinae muscle group, which consists of four separate but intertwined muscles. They are the iliocostalis thoracis, the iliocostalis lumborum, the longissimus dorsi, and the spinalis dorsi. These muscles have the same action and work in conjunction with one another. Together, these long, slender muscles cover a large area running from the neck to the sacrum directly on the posterior spine and on both sides of the spine. When the erector spinae is well developed (hypertrophied), a groove can be seen between the left and right sides.

More specifically, these superficial muscles originate on the crest of the ilium, the lower surface of the sacrum, the borders of the lower seven ribs, the spinous processes of all the lumbar and the lower four thoracic vertebrae, and the transverse processes of all the thoracic vertebrae. Muscle insertion is on the angles of the ribs and on the transverse processes of all the vertebrae.

The deep spinal muscle group (not shown) is comprised of the intertransversarii, interspinalis, rotatores, and multifidus muscles, which are very small and run in pairs. These muscles join the transverse and spinous processes of adjacent vertebrae. Most often they attach only to the vertebrae next to them, but some may extend over two or three vertebrae. They play an important role in holding the vertebrae and discs in place as well as in moving the spine.

The erector spinae and the deep spinal muscles are involved in extension and hyperextension of the lower spine. In this action you raise the upper trunk up and back until your body forms a straight line. The axis of rotation is in the waist.

Lateral flexion of the spine involves the abdominals, the erector spinae, and the quadratus lumborum. The major muscles involved are the quadratus lumborum, the abdominal obliques, and the erector spinae. The quadratus lumborum is a flat sheet of deep muscle fibers located on each side of the spinal column (see Figure 6.2).

The origin of the quadratus lumborum is on the crest of the ilium and the ligament and

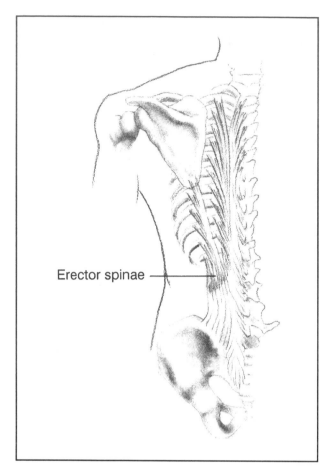

Figure 6.1
The back: superficial spinal muscles

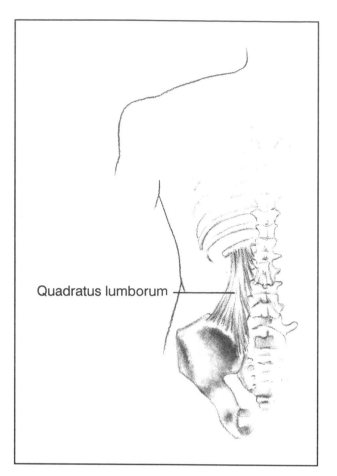

Figure 6.2
Posterior view of the back

transverse processes of the lower four lumbar vertebrae. Insertion is on the transverse processes of the upper two lumbar vertebrae and the lower border of the last rib.

When lateral flexion occurs as, for example, when you lie on your side, the upper half of the erector spinae and the upper half of the rectus abdominis, the upper quadratus lumborum, and the internal and external obliques are involved. Forward spinal rotation involves the abdominals, whereas backward spinal rotation involves the erector spinae.

■ Back Raise

The back raise is the only exercise in which the lower back spinal muscles can be worked through a full range of motion in a very safe manner. I developed this exercise several years

ago after looking closely at the spinal musculature and asking why hyperextensions did not exercise the area safely and effectively. Since then, the back raise has been used very successfully by athletes and non-athletes in the treatment and prevention of back problems.

Major muscles and actions involved

In back raises the erector spinae and the deep back muscles are involved in extension–hyperextension (see Figure 6.3). In this action the trunk is raised to the horizontal position from an inverted vertical hanging position.

Sports uses

The erector spinae muscle is important in most sports, even though it may not directly participate in moving the spine in extension or hyperextension. It must be strong enough to hold the vertebrae (spine) in place and rigid when you

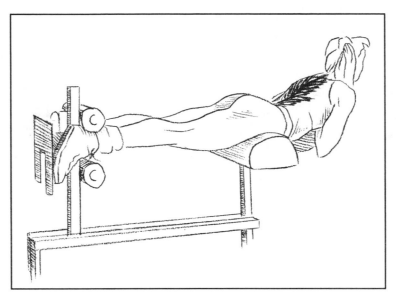

Figure 6.3
Muscles used in the back raise

execute many skills, especially those involved in lifting. For example, the erectors are most important in keeping the spine in lordosis during the squat, good morning, and deadlift exercises.

The sports of wrestling (wrestler bridge), gymnastics, diving, and ballet (to assume correct posture and to straighten the body from a tucked position) involve a great deal of extension and hyperextension of the spine. Many take-downs and throws in the sports of judo and wrestling rely upon extension and hyperextension of the spine. Rowers need strong erectors for pulling the oars, and cyclists need them to keep their backs from getting sore when they ride in the racing position.

The spinal extensors play an important role in all sports that require jumping, for example, the high jump, pole vault, basketball, and volleyball. Football and ice hockey players need strong erectors to withstand blows to the body, whereas golfers and tennis, baseball, and racquetball players require strong backs to do the necessary twisting, bending, and reaching needed in their sports.

The erector spinae muscles are important for many more sports that could be listed here, but it is simpler to say that without development of these muscles, most athletes are likely to experience back problems. The key value of the development of these muscles is not to enhance

particular sports actions, but to make it possible for other actions to take place and to prevent injury.

Execution

Back raises are most conveniently and safely done on a BFS Glute-Ham Developer (GHD). If you do not have a GHD available to you, you can use a sturdy table and an assistant. To position yourself, lie in a prone position over the curved seat of the GHD so that when your feet are secured between the rear pads your entire pelvic girdle rests on the seat. Hang your upper trunk over the seat, keeping your spinal muscles relaxed. In this position, your spine will naturally assume a rounded position and will be at approximately a 60-degree angle below the horizontal. Your legs should be fully extended and kept straight at all times (see Photo 6.1).

From this position, inhale slightly more than usual and hold your breath as you extend (straighten) your spine. Raise your head and the thoracic portion of your spine first and then raise your trunk. Raise your upper trunk until it is slightly higher than your legs, i.e., arched (see Photo 6.2). After reaching the uppermost position, exhale and return to the initial position under control. When you reach the lowermost position, relax your muscles and then repeat.

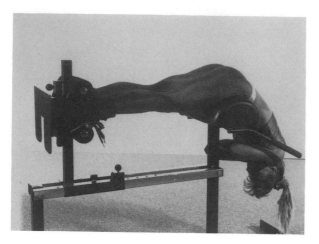

Photo 6.1

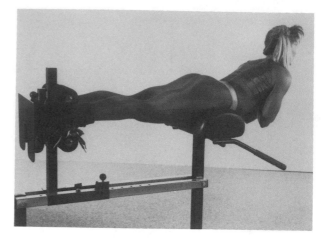

Photo 6.2

Comments

- When you do this exercise, it is important to have your spine rounded as much as possible before you begin the upward extension movement. This will stretch the muscles and provide for a stronger contraction. It will also allow for a good stretch of the spine (the vertebrae are pulled apart). Thus, when you rise up, you develop the muscles from an elongated position. This is especially important in rehabilitation.

- Back raises, and even hyperextensions, have been criticized as being dangerous because of the arching of the spine. However, it is important to understand that the arched position is normal—a healthy, strong spine is arched in the lumbar area in the neutral position. Problems occur only when the arching is excessive or when your spine is kept in a flexed position most of the time. Even more importantly, if you keep your legs straight throughout the entire execution of this exercise, it is impossible to arch (hyperextend) your spine excessively. In the arching that may occur, the muscles are responsible for the action and they hold the spine in place to prevent injury.

- If you bend your knees as you do this exercise, your trunk becomes more upright where the compression forces are greater, and hyperextension can occur. This can be dangerous. Also, when hyperextension occurs with gravity as the moving force (as when doing a back arch from a standing position), the spinal muscles are relaxed and stress falls on the vertebrae

and discs. Such movements can also cause injury.

- When you execute the back raise, it is extremely important to have your pelvic girdle situated on the seat of the Glute-Ham Developer. Your navel should be in line with the far edge of the seat or slightly ahead of it. A Roman chair or hyperextension bench can be used for execution of the back raise if you duplicate this position on them. However, in this exercise, remember that when your feet are in place, your pelvis is on the seat. For most people, this is not possible when they use a Roman chair unless they place their calves under the leg retainers, which can hurt the muscles. A safe alternative is to use a high, sturdy bench and have someone hold down your legs. Execution is then the same. However, in this variant you should place a rolled-up towel under your lower abdomen to help increase intra-abdominal pressure.

- If your pelvic girdle is allowed to extend beyond the seat, the axis of rotation switches to your hips, and the hip joint extensor muscles (gluteus maximus and hamstrings) come into play. This is the positioning used to do the hyperextension. When this positioning occurs, however, there is a tendency to "snap" the trunk upward with spinal extension-hyperextension as hip joint extension takes place. This action can be injurious! In fact, it is because of this that the hyperextension exercise has been severely criticized. The key to safety when doing hyperextensions is to maintain your spine in a rigid arched position throughout the execution.

■ Back Raise with a Twist

Many athletes, bodybuilders, and fitness buffs think that trunk rotation is a function of the abdominals. This is true to a large extent, but only when the movement is in a forward direction. When you twist backwards, which occurs not only in many sports but in many common everyday activities, you use the erector spinae of the lower back. Thus, to fully develop this muscle, you can do the back raise with a twist exercise.

Major muscles and actions involved

The same as for the back raise.

Sports uses

In addition to the sports uses listed in the section on the back raise, it should be mentioned that the twisting movement can give an even a greater range of motion in trunk rotation in throwing and hitting actions. Developing the rotational action of these muscles helps to provide greater stability in the midsection.

Execution

Back raises with a twist are executed in the same way as back raises, but with the following differences: When you are in the down position, place an Exer Stick (or long pole) across your shoulders and hold it in place with your arms outstretched (see Photo 6.3). If you have great flexibility in your waist, you may find that the handles of the GHD hit your arms. To avoid this, do not go down to the lowest position but remain slightly above the handles.

When you are ready, inhale and hold your breath as you raise your trunk up to the horizontal or slightly above horizontal position and then rotate up to 90 degrees to one side so that your trunk and arms form the letter T (see Photo 6.4). Return to the face-down position and lower yourself to the initial position, exhaling as you do so. After a momentary pause, inhale again and raise your trunk. When your body is horizontal, rotate up to 90 degrees to the opposite side. Turn back to the face-down position, lower your body, and then repeat, twisting to alternate sides.

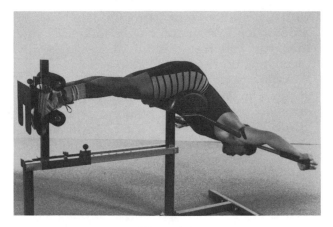

Photo 6.3

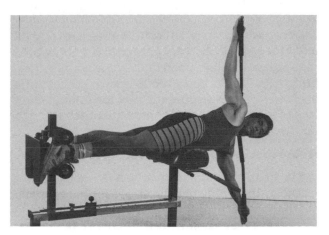

Photo 6.4

Comments

- The main value of this exercise lies in the twisting, and therefore it is not important that you go to the lowermost position. When you are advanced and can hold yourself horizontally, you can then twist alternately to the right and left while maintaining your body in a straight position, similar to the Russian twist. However, for most people it is most convenient to do a back raise together with the twisting.

- You can use either a long, straight pole or an Exer Stick to do this exercise. The Exer Stick is preferred, however, because it has a curvature in the middle of the pole which fits comfortably around your neck area and keeps the pole directly in line with your shoulders and arms. If you use a pole, the pole must be long enough to keep your arms out in a straight line with your shoulders. (Do not use a short broomstick.) When you have a long lever like this, you can rotate more easily, especially through a full range of motion.

- You will notice in doing this exercise that your gluteus maximus and hamstrings will be strongly contracted to stabilize your pelvic girdle. For greater stabilization, it is important to keep your pelvic girdle directly on the seat. If your pelvic girdle extends over the seat, then part of the rotation will be in the hip joints rather than isolated in the waist.

◼ Back Extension on a Back Exercise Machine

Because the axis of rotation of most back machines is closer to the hips than the waist, these machines are used mainly for stabilization purposes. When you execute exercises using a back exercise machine, the erector spinae muscles of your lower back contract isometrically to hold your spine in place.

Major muscles and actions involved

The erector spinae is involved isometrically to stabilize the spine. In the hip joint the gluteus maximus and the upper hamstrings are involved in hip joint extension (see Figure 6.4). In this action the trunk moves backward with the axis in the hip joint.

Sports uses

Stabilization of the spine is very important in all lifting exercises. When the spine is stabilized, it is held in its proper shape while some activity is done, for example, a squat or overhead press. Some individuals, often inadvisably, use their backs when they lift weights off the floor, especially if they lack flexibility in their hip joints or do not have the strength to hold their spines rigid. Thus, in bodybuilding, as well as many other sports, the erector spinae and the spinal extension actions are not usually stressed, and as a result, many bodybuilders have weak lower backs. Development of these muscles, however, can add much to total back strength and definition. Spinal stabilization is very important in the prevention of back injuries, and it plays a role in many different sports and occupations. Because of this, machine back extensions should be a part of your exercise arsenal.

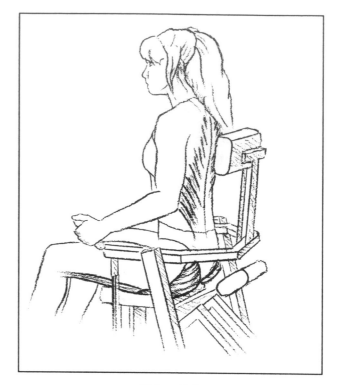

Figure 6.4
Muscles used in back extension (machine)

Execution

Because of its greater versatility and safety, the Keiser back machine will be described. For proper positioning, sit down on the machine in an erect position and place your pelvis against the lower pelvis cushion. When this is done, your hips are properly positioned and you become aligned with the machine's pivot axis. Strap your pelvis in to prevent excess motion, and place your feet against the adjustable footrests to accommodate your leg length (see Photo 6.5). Decrease the resistance with the hand buttons so that the back lever arm is free to move with no resistance.

With your trunk erect and placed against the back lever arm, increase the resistance to the necessary tension on the muscles. Then inhale and hold your breath as you push back through approximately a 60-degree range of motion (see Photo 6.6). Relax your muscles slightly and return to the initial position or even farther to the front, depending upon your flexibility. Exhale as you approach the forward position and then repeat. Keep your spine in basically the

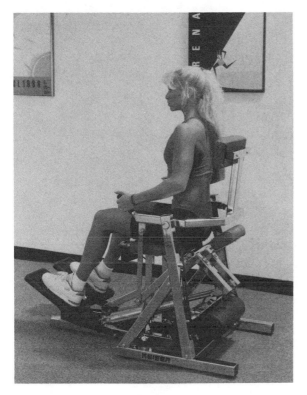

Photo 6.5

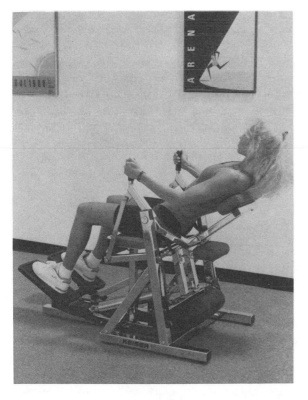

Photo 6.6

same normal anatomical position throughout the execution.

To avoid injury, do back extensions slowly or at a moderate rate of speed. Be conscious of the actions taking place. Do not do any quick or snapping movements, especially if they involve flexing or extending the lumbar area of your spine.

Comments

- In seated back machine exercises, the main action is in your hip joint. Your lower back remains basically rigid to push the resistance bar backward. Because of this, the erector spinae muscles of your back remain in isometric contraction in their stabilizing action. Your gluteus maximus and upper hamstrings are, however, dynamically contracting to move your trunk backwards.

- Physiological studies indicate that strength can be developed from either a concentric or isometric contraction. However, the concentric contraction, in which the muscle shortens and the bony attachments move, is much more effective. Also, the isometric contraction, in which the muscle fibers shorten somewhat but there is no movement, develops strength only at the point in which the body or limbs are held. Thus, in this exercise the back muscles are developed with the trunk held in basically the anatomical position.

- Because you are sitting down when you do this exercise, you should immediately try to straighten or slightly arch your back if you start with a flexed back. (On the Keiser machine this is done very easily by completely removing the resistance.) You should then keep your back in a lordotic (arched) position as you push back. Do not excessively hyperextend your spine. When you push back and arch a great deal, especially if the resistance is very great, you can create compression and shearing forces on the vertebrae and discs. This, in turn, can cause an injury.

- Also, you should be careful not to arch your back excessively if you already have swayback (an excessively arched lumbar spine). If you arch back all the way (as is possible on some machines), you can accentuate the swayback condition, which can bring on or increase the pressure on the discs and nerves. This, in turn, will cause or increase back pain.

• Exercising the back muscles (the erector spinae) is a relatively new phenomenon in the United States. For many years it was believed that it was only necessary to strengthen the abdominals and stretch the back in order to strengthen the spine. But today strengthening the erector spinae muscles is known to be as effective, if not more so, for the development of a strong, healthy spine. Thus, you should use some type of back strengthening exercise to prevent injury and enhance your performance of many activities.

■ Side Bend

Side bends involve not only all of the abdominal and lower back muscles, but also the quadratus lumborum. A key back muscle, the quadratus lumborum is very important in lateral stability of the spine. The only exercise that involves this muscle is the side bend and its several variants.

Major muscles and actions involved

In side bends the quadratus lumborum, the internal and external obliques, the rectus abdominis, and the erector spinae muscles are involved in lateral flexion of the spine (see Figures 6.5, 6.6, and 6.7). In this action the trunk is pulled over to one side.

Sports uses

This exercise is important for all athletes who throw overhead for maximum distance or force (baseball pitchers, outfielders, football quarterbacks, javelin throwers). It is also important for overhead hitting (tennis serve and smash, racquetball ceiling shot, badminton overhead clear and smash) and when you reach up as high as possible (basketball rebounding, volleyball spike, catching fly balls).

The side bend exercise is very valuable for gymnasts performing on the pommel horse, horizontal bar (unevens), and in free exercise (cartwheels and other similar movements in the lateral plane). In addition, it is needed by acrobats for many stunts and hand balances, modern and ballet dancers, divers, and trampolinists. The movements in this exercise play a role in punch-

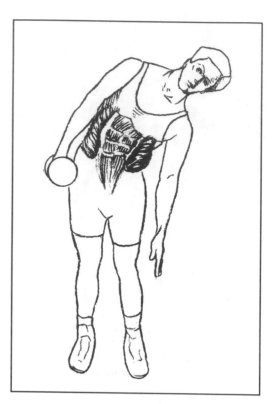

Figure 6.5
Muscles used in the standing side bend
(Variant 1)

ing in karate and boxing, in kicking in the martial arts, and in many wrestling activities.

Bodybuilders and athletes need this exercise for maximum development of the abdominal and low back musculature. This exercise is also very valuable for all athletes who must do heavy lifting overhead or who receive heavy blows to the body from the side, as in football. In essence, it is valuable for maintaining good posture and a strong midsection.

Execution

There are three major variants of the side bend.

Variant 1—*Standing side bend:* Stand up and hold a dumbbell in one hand. Your other hand can be left alongside your body or placed behind your head. Keep your weight equally balanced on both your feet, and keep your pelvic girdle firmly in place at all times (see Photo 6.7).

When you are ready, lower your shoulders and upper trunk to the same side as the dumbbell as far as possible without shifting your pelvis to the

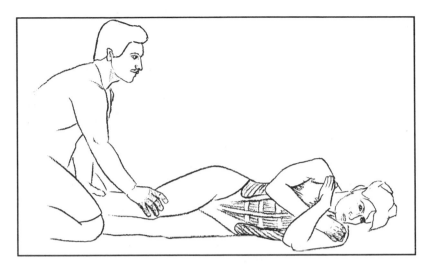

Figure 6.6
Muscles used in the floor side bend
(Variant 2)

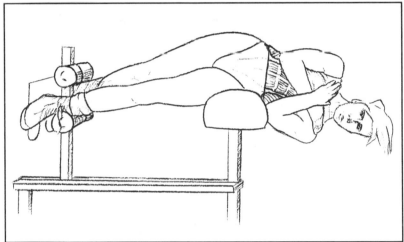

Figure 6.7
Muscles used in the GHD side bend
(Variant 3)

other side (see Photo 6.8). Upon reaching the bottom position, inhale and hold your breath as you raise your trunk sideways back to the erect standing position and over to the other side as far as possible (see Photo 6.9). Exhale as you reach the vertical. Pause momentarily and then repeat.

Variant 2—*Floor side bend:* Lie on your side on the floor and have an assistant sit on your feet and place his or her hands on your upper thighs or hips to keep them in place. Cross your hands on your chest and keep your head aligned with your trunk (see Photo 6.10.) When you are ready, inhale slightly more than usual and hold your breath as you raise your trunk sideways as high as possible (see Photo 6.11). Be sure that your trunk remains in the side plane at all times. When reaching the uppermost position, exhale and return to the original position, keeping your

body under control. Pause momentarily and then repeat.

Variant 3—*Glute-Ham Developer side bend:* To increase the range of motion and the intensity of the muscular contractions, do this exercise on the Glute-Ham Developer. Position yourself sideways on the Glute-Ham Developer with your hips directly on the seat. Your trunk will be unsupported and held in place in a horizontal position by your midsection muscles. Then lower your trunk under control as far as possible so that your muscles are placed on maximum stretch (see Photo 6.12). After you have reached the bottom position, raise your trunk up as high as possible so that your trunk goes through approximately a 90-degree range of motion (see Photo 6.13). In this variant you do forced breathing. Exhale quickly and then inhale and hold your breath as you lower and raise your trunk.

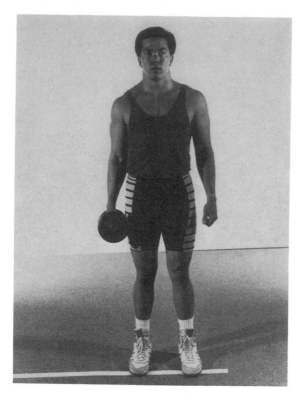

Photo 6.7

Comments

- When executed correctly, the side bend exercise is relatively difficult to execute (except for the standing position variant). The muscles involved in this exercise are very often weak for this action because people generally exercise only in the anterior-posterior plane (from back to front), not in the lateral plane.

- The usual range of motion in this exercise is not great. The maximum appears to be 30–45 degrees on one side. Therefore, if you are not extremely flexible and you find yourself going through a range of motion greater than 45 degrees, you are most likely moving your hips to increase the range of motion.

- When you execute the side bend exercise from a standing position, your pelvic girdle must be stabilized by your hip joint muscles. When lateral flexion occurs, your upper body moves down mainly due to gravity; your upper body rises due to the actions of the internal and external obliques, the quadratus lumborum, and the erector spinae and rectus abdominis on the opposite side (the side to which you are moving).

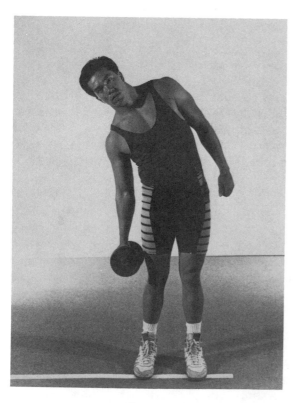

Photo 6.8

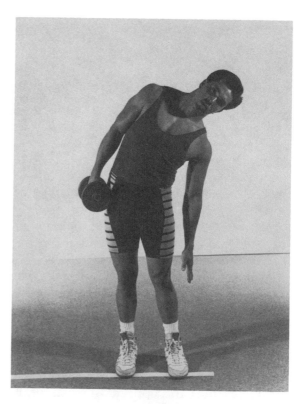

Photo 6.9

When you do the exercise on the Glute-Ham Developer or lying on the floor, it also involves all the muscles on one side. However, execution on the Glute-Ham Developer is much more effective because it allows for a greater range of motion, which gives greater development to the muscles. It is important to understand that this is the only exercise in which your trunk is pulled from the opposite side (below the horizontal) through the same side as the muscles involved.

- The quadratus lumborum is a major muscle involved in this movement because lateral flexion is its only action. Development of this muscle is needed for lateral stability of the spine and in preventing the spine from curving to the left or right, which results in scoliosis.

Because the quadratus lumborum is a deep muscle, it cannot be felt or seen, but it is critical to a safe and pain-free lower back.

- To help ensure that you have proper isolation of the muscles involved, remain in the lateral plane during exercise execution. Do not rotate your trunk or hips to the right or left prior to or during the action. Doing this brings other muscles into play but, more importantly, it can cause injury.

- Additional resistance is not needed when you are first beginning this exercise except in the standing variant, which requires the use of a dumbbell. For the other variants, the weight of your upper body is quite sufficient. If you can execute the exercise easily, you should then hold light weights in your hands on your chest.

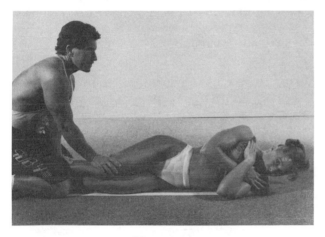

Photo 6.10

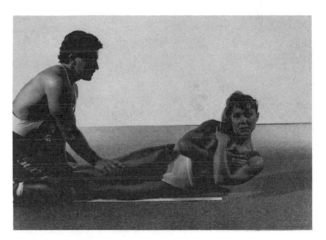

Photo 6.11

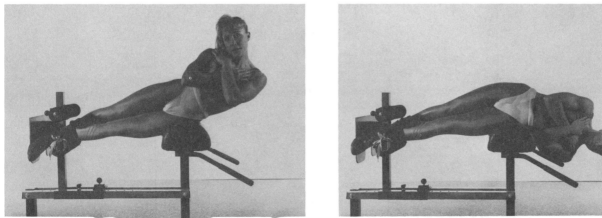

Photo 6.12   Photo 6.13

■ Reverse Back Raise

An effective variant of the back raise exercise, which I developed, is called the reverse back raise. This exercise is the opposite of the back raise, just as the reverse sit-up is the opposite of the sit-up. It is best suited for people who cannot hang upside down, and it can also be used for variety.

Major muscles and actions involved

In the reverse back raise the erector spinae muscle of the lower back is involved in spinal extension–hyperextension (see Figure 6.8). In this action you raise your hips and legs from a vertical hanging position up to the horizontal or slightly above. The axis of rotation is in the waist.

Sports uses

The same as for the back raise.

Execution

This exercise is most effectively done on a BFS Glute-Ham Developer, but it is also possible to use a high, sturdy, relatively narrow table. The description for the GHD will be given because of its greater ease of execution and effectiveness.

Face the GHD from the seated end. Lean over the rounded seat so that your lower abdomen and pelvis are supported on the far side of the curved seat. Grasp the rollers or back plate with your hands to secure your head and shoulders in place. Your feet should be hanging down at approximately a 30-degree angle to the vertical (see Photo 6.14). When you are ready, hold tight with your hands and then inhale and hold your breath as you raise your pelvis and legs as a unit. In the ending position your legs and pelvis should be slightly higher than the level of your back (see Photo 6.15). After reaching the upper-most position, exhale and return to the initial position. Pause for a moment and then repeat.

Comments

- For proper execution it is important that you hold on tightly with your hands to hold your upper body in place. The same applies to doing the exercise on a high, sturdy table. By holding your upper trunk in place, you can isolate the action of the erector spinae when raising your pelvis and legs as a unit.

- It is also important that you position yourself properly so that your hips hang over the rounded seat. If you position yourself with your hips directly on top of the seat with only your feet hanging over, you will be working only the gluteus maximus and upper hamstrings in hip joint extension. The erector spinae would not come into play then until you

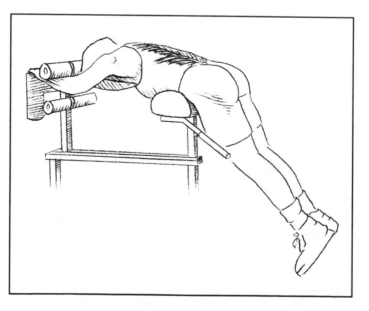

Figure 6.8
Muscles used in the reverse back raise

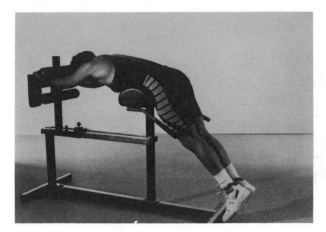

Photo 6.14

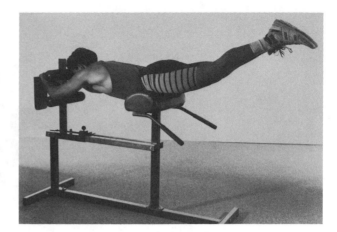

Photo 6.15

raised your legs higher than the horizontal position.

■ Additional Exercises for the Lower Back Muscles

There are other common exercises for the erector spinae, but they either do not go through a full range of motion or they are used mainly in rehabilitation. For example, the pelvic thrust is one of the most effective yet simple exercises that can be done at home. To do this exercise, lie flat on the floor with your knees bent, your feet flat on the floor, and your arms alongside your body. Then raise your trunk until your body forms a straight line (or arched back) between your knees and shoulders (see Photo 6.16). Do not confuse this exercise with the pelvic tilt (an abdominal exercise) in which you rotate your pelvis backward in an attempt to flatten your back.

The floor arch exercise is effective for a short ending range of motion. To execute the floor arch, lie face down on the floor and then raise your trunk and legs as high as possible, although this will not be very high (see Photo 6.17). If this version is too difficult, you can raise only your legs or only your trunk.

For stabilization of the spine, you can do the cross-body lift. To execute, get down on all fours so that there is a right angle between your arms and trunk and your thighs and trunk. When you are ready, inhale and raise one arm and the

opposite leg until they are in line with or slightly above the level of your back (see Photo 6.18). Return to the initial position and repeat with the opposite arm and leg. If you raise your arm and leg beyond the normal arched position of the spine, you will also be involving the erector spinae dynamically.

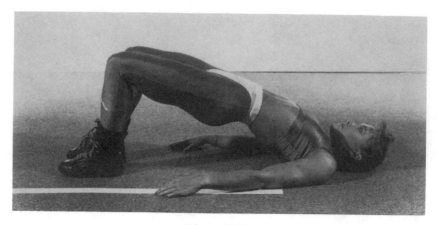

Photo 6.16

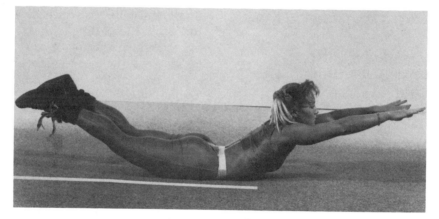

Photo 6.17

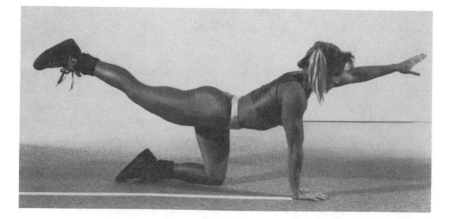

Photo 6.18

PART THREE

The Upper Body

7 The Shoulder Joint

ANATOMY OF THE SHOULDER JOINT AND SHOULDER GIRDLE

The shoulder joint is the most freely movable of all the body's ball-and-socket joints. Because of this, the greatest variety and combination of movements at a joint can be executed by the arm from the shoulder joint.

The shoulder joint is formed by the articulation of the glenoid fossa of the scapula (shoulder blade) and the head of the humerus (upper arm bone). The shoulder joint consists of a shallow socket (glenoid cavity) into which the half-spherical head of the humerus fits. It should be noted that less than half of the humerus is in the socket at any time. Because of this, the bony arrangement is very weak and therefore the strength of the musculature around the shoulder is very important for stability.

It is impossible to talk about the movements of the shoulder joint without also discussing the shoulder girdle, which consists of the scapula and clavicle (collar bone). The clavicle joins the sternum (breast bone) at the sternoclavicular joint, which allows for full-range movement of the outer (shoulder) end of the clavicle. The outer end of the clavicle joins the scapula at the acromion in what is known as the acromioclavicular joint.

Because the clavicle cannot move by itself, movements of the shoulder girdle are usually referred to as movements of the scapula, which is free to move in all directions. Thus, scapula movements allow for a greatly increased range of motion in the shoulder joint by changing the position of the joint.

BASIC MOVEMENTS IN THE SHOULDER JOINT AND SHOULDER GIRDLE

The movements possible in the shoulder joint are as follows: flexion, in which the arm is moved upward and in front; the return movement is known as extension, in which the arm moves down and to the rear; and hyperextension, when the arm passes the plane of the body and continues moving backward and upward.

When your arm is raised overhead, not only does your arm move up, but your scapula rotates upward as well. Without this movement of the scapula, it would be impossible to raise your arms above the level of your shoulders. In upward rotation of the scapula, the upper end of the scapula moves closer to the spine and the lower end moves out to the sides of the body along the ribs. For simplicity's sake, it can be said that when viewed from the rear, in upward rotation of the scapulae, the right scapula rotates counterclockwise and the left scapula rotates clockwise on an axis through the center of the scapulae.

In extension the scapulae rotate downward in synchronization with the arms. In this movement the actions are the reverse of upward rotation, that is, the right scapula rotates clockwise and the left scapula rotates counterclockwise on an axis through the center of the scapulae.

Movement of the arm sideward and upward is known as abduction, and the return movement with the arm moving sideward and downward toward the body is known as adduction. To allow the arm to move sideward and upward through a full range of motion, the scapula must also undergo upward rotation the same as in shoulder flexion. In adduction the same actions occur as in shoulder extension.

The movement of the arm as it moves horizontally toward the front of the body is known as horizontal flexion or horizontal adduction. Movement in the opposite direction, from the front position horizontally to the side, is known as horizontal extension or horizontal abduction.

In these actions the scapulae must also provide a full range of motion. In horizontal adduction with the arms moving to the front, the scapulae abduct. In this action they slide out along the rib cage toward the sides of the body. In horizontal abduction when the arms are moving toward the rear, the scapulae adduct, that is, move inward toward the spine.

The humerus can also be turned inward around its long axis, which is known as medial or inward rotation. Outward or lateral rotation is the opposite movement, in which the arm rotates to the outside. In medial and lateral rotation the scapula does not rotate if the movement is done through a normal range of motion. When the movement is beyond a normal range of motion, the scapula is forced into movement that is not normal for it, and this can lead to injury.

It is also possible to elevate and depress the shoulder girdle. In this case the entire shoulder girdle (clavicle and scapula) is raised upward in an action called shoulder girdle elevation; lowering the shoulder girdle is called shoulder girdle depression.

MAJOR MUSCLES INVOLVED IN THE SHOULDER JOINT

Movements of the shoulder joint are produced by 11 muscles. Two of these muscles (the biceps brachii and triceps brachii) have only assisting actions in the shoulder joint because their major action is at the elbow joint. The main muscles

are the deltoid, supraspinatus, pectoralis major, coracobrachialis, latissimus dorsi, teres major, infraspinatus, teres minor, and subscapularis.

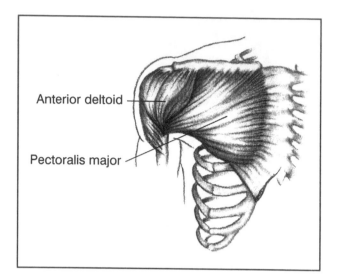

Figure 7.1
Anterior view of the chest (right side)

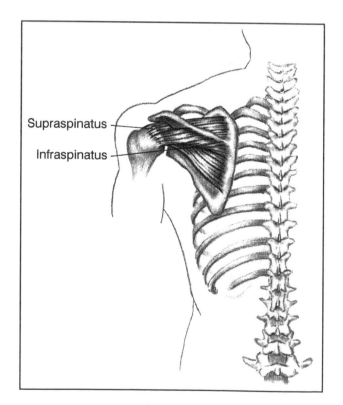

Figure 7.2
Posterior view (deep) of the left shoulder

100

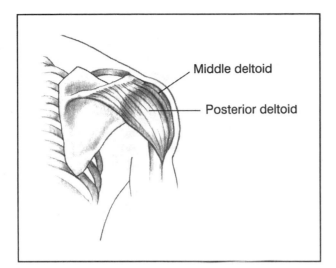

Figure 7.3
Posterior view of the right shoulder

Shoulder joint abduction

The major muscles involved in shoulder joint abduction are the deltoid and the supraspinatus (see Figures 7.1, 7.2, and 7.3). The deltoid has three distinct sections—the anterior, middle, and posterior portions, which cover the front, top, and rear of the shoulder respectively. The deltoid originates on the outer third of the clavicle, the top of the acromion, and the posterior border of the scapular spine, and it inserts on the deltoid tuberosity of the humerus (just above the center of the bone).

The supraspinatus lies under the deltoid in the supraspinatus fossa on the top posterior section of the scapula (see Figure 7.2). More specifically, it originates on the inner two-thirds of the supraspinatus fossa and inserts on the top of the greater tubercle of the humerus (the top outside portion of the head of the humerus).

Shoulder joint adduction

The major muscles involved in shoulder joint adduction are the latissimus dorsi, the teres major, and the lower pectoralis major.

The latissimus dorsi covers a very wide area of the lower half and upper sides of the back. It originates on the spinous processes of the lower thoracic and all the lumbar vertebrae, the back of the sacrum, the crest of the ilium, and the lower three ribs. It inserts on the upper anterior side of the humerus by a flat tendon attached

parallel to the upper portion of the pectoralis major insertion (see Figure 7.4).

The teres major is located on the upper sides of the back. It is a round muscle which originates on the lower end of the lateral border of the scapula and inserts on the upper anterior portion of the humerus parallel to and slightly lower than the insertion of the latissimus dorsi (see Figure 7.4).

Horizontal adduction

In this action, also known as horizontal flexion, the major muscles are the pectoralis major, the coracobrachialis, and the anterior deltoid.

The pectoralis major originates on the anterior border of the clavicle, the entire length of the sternum, and the cartilages of the first six ribs near the sternum. It inserts by a flat tendon

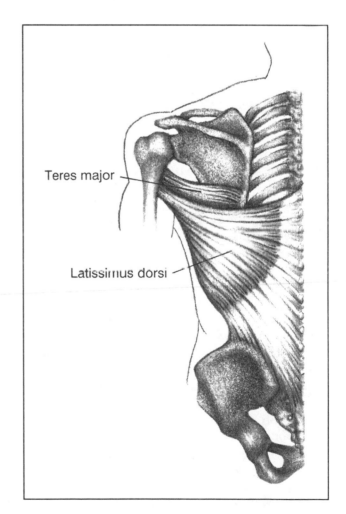

Figure 7.4
Posterior view of the back (left side)

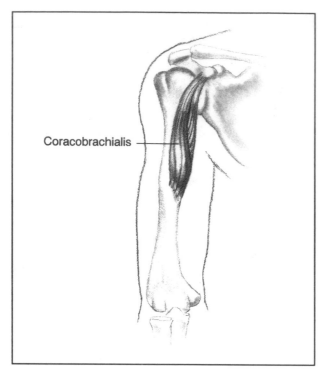

Figure 7.5
Anterior view of the upper right arm

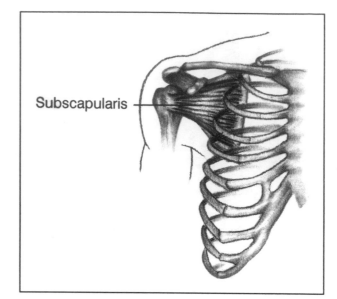

Figure 7.6
Anterior view of the right chest

to the outer lip of the intertubercular groove of the humerus nearly down to the insertion of the deltoid (see Figure 7.1).

The coracobrachialis is a small muscle located deep underneath the deltoid and pectoralis major muscles. It originates on the coracoid process of the scapula and inserts on the inner front surface of the humerus just opposite the deltoid (see Figure 7.5).

It is interesting to note the structure of the latissimus dorsi and pectoralis major muscles, especially their tendons of insertion. As the latissimus dorsi crosses the shoulder joint, its fibers twist around so that the anterior fibers become posterior and the posterior fibers become anterior. The pectoralis major muscle fibers also do a 180-degree twist so that where the muscle inserts on the humerus, the lower fibers are uppermost and the upper fibers are lowermost. This twisting of the muscle fibers prior to insertion makes possible the many different actions that these muscles are capable of (shoulder joint flexion, extension, medial rotation, adduction, and horizontal adduction by the pectoralis major; and extension, inward rotation, adduction,

horizontal abduction, and hyperextension by the latissimus dorsi).

Horizontal abduction

In this action, also known as horizontal extension, the major muscles involved are the middle and posterior deltoid, the infraspinatus, and the teres minor (see Figures 7.2 and 7.3). The infraspinatus originates on the infraspinatus fossa of the scapula and inserts on the greater tubercle of the humerus. The teres minor originates on the dorsal surface of the lateral border of the scapula and inserts on the lower portion of the greater tubercle just below the infraspinatus.

Shoulder joint flexion

The anterior deltoid, the pectoralis major (upper portion), and the coracobrachialis are the major muscles involved in shoulder joint flexion.

Shoulder joint extension

This action is the opposite of shoulder joint flexion. The major muscles involved are the middle and posterior deltoid, the teres minor, and the infraspinatus.

Inward rotation

In this action, also known as medial rotation, the major muscles involved are the subscapularis, the latissimus dorsi, and the teres major. The subscapularis originates on the entire costal surface of the scapula and inserts on the lesser tubercle of the humerus (see Figure 7.6).

Outward rotation

In this action, also known as lateral rotation, the major muscles involved are the infraspinatus and the teres minor.

MAJOR MUSCLES INVOLVED IN THE SHOULDER GIRDLE

The trapezius is a large, flat sheet of muscle located on the upper and middle portion of the back. It originates on the base of the skull, the ligament of the neck, and the spinous processes of the 7th cervical to the 12th thoracic vertebrae. It inserts along a curved line on the outer third of the posterior border of the clavicle, the top of the acromium, and the upper border of the spine of the scapula (see Figure 7.7). The middle fibers of the trapezius are involved in scapula adduc-

tion. They work together with the rhomboid in pulling the scapula in close to the spine.

The very uppermost portion of the trapezius is involved in scapula elevation. Assisting it is the levator scapulae muscle. The levator scapulae is a small muscle on the back and side of the neck beneath the upper trapezius. It runs from the transverse processes of the upper four or five cervical vertebrae to the medial border of the scapula (see Figure 7.7).

Just below the very top portion of the trapezius, the fibers of the trapezius begin to run in a more diagonal fashion. These upper fibers are involved in upward rotation of the scapula. The lower fibers of the trapezius also have a downward pull on the inside edge of the scapula so that they too are involved in upward rotation. The serratus anterior also pulls on the outer bottom portion of the scapula for upward rotation.

The rhomboid lies beneath the middle of the trapezius. It originates on the spinous processes of the upper thoracic vertebrae and inserts on the medial border of the scapula (see Figure 7.8). It has two major actions: scapula adduction and downward rotation. The direction that the fibers run in the rhomboid makes the muscle ideally suited for downward rotation.

The serratus anterior lies on the outer surface of the ribs at the side and is covered by the

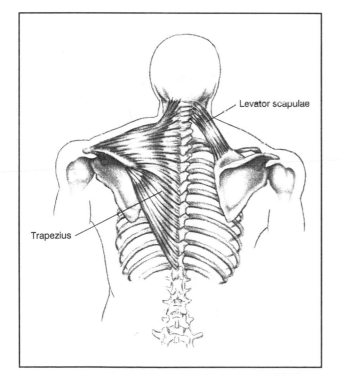

Figure 7.7
Posterior view of the back

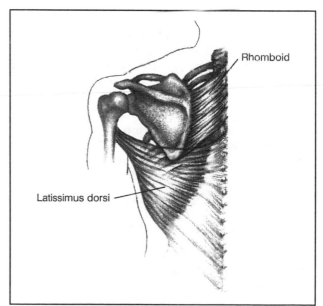

Figure 7.8
Posterior view of the back (left side)

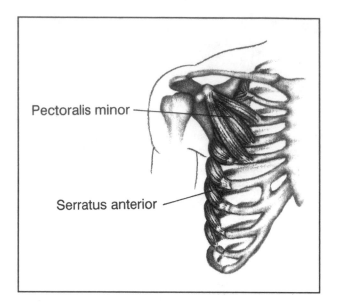

Figure 7.9
Anterior view of the chest (right side)

scapula at the rear and the pectoralis major in front. It originates on the outer surfaces of the upper eight or nine ribs at the side of the chest in between the attachments of the external oblique. It inserts on the anterior surface of the medial border of the scapula (see Figure 7.9). The serratus anterior is involved in upward rotation of the scapula and in abduction, that is, it helps pull the scapula to the sides away from the spine.

The pectoralis minor is a small muscle located on the front of the upper chest that is covered by the pectoralis major. It runs from the outer surfaces of the third, fourth, and fifth ribs at one end and is attached to the end of the coracoid at the other end (see Figure 7.9).

The pectoralis minor is involved in depression and abduction. In depression it works together with the lower trapezius, and in abduction it works together with the serratus anterior.

SHOULDER JOINT EXERCISES

■ Front Arm Raise

In many sports and occupations, most of the body's movement takes place in front of the body. The front arm raise can be done to en-

hance some of these movements and to maintain or even improve flexibility.

Major muscles and actions involved

The anterior deltoid, the pectoralis major (upper portion), and the coracobrachialis are involved in the front arm raise (see Figure 7.10). The action is shoulder joint flexion, in which the arms move directly forward and upward from a position alongside the body. In the shoulder girdle the serratus anterior and the upper and lower trapezius are involved in upward rotation of the scapula. When both arms are involved, the right scapula rotates counterclockwise and the left rotates clockwise on an axis through the center of each bone. When only one arm is used, the scapula also usually undergoes abduction, in which it moves away from the spine toward the sides of the rib cage.

Sports uses

Shoulder joint flexion and the muscles involved are most important in sports that require

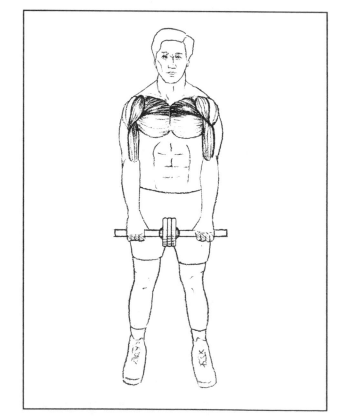

Figure 7.10
Muscles used in the front arm raise

you to move your arms up and in front, such as gymnastics and diving, and in basketball and volleyball when you reach upward to get or block the ball. They are also needed in boxing to get the arm up and in the uppercut; and in judo, wrestling, and other sports. However, most often these movements are not done against a heavy resistance.

The muscles and arm action used in the front arm raise are very important to football linemen when blocking or hitting an opponent. They are also used in underhand throwing and hitting actions, as, for example, in bowling and softball pitching and in underhand shots in the racquet sports and handball. They are important in raising the bat in baseball, the cross in lacrosse, and the hockey stick in hockey in preparation for different shots.

For bodybuilders, this exercise is very important in developing the uppermost front portions of the shoulders and chest. It gives fullness to the upper chest. Also, this exercise is very important in preventing injuries to the shoulder joint and middle upper back.

Execution

The front arm raise can be done with a barbell, dumbbells, or a Strength Bar. With a barbell, because the weights are placed on the ends, the stress of the weight is distributed fairly equally on the shoulders. Dumbbells are more versatile and enable you to do the exercise either unilaterally or in an alternating fashion. However, to place greater stress on the anterior deltoid, the Strength Bar is preferred. The Strength Bar is a relatively short bar with the weights located in the middle and concentrated directly in front of the body. The front arm raise exercise will be described using a Strength Bar, but the basic execution is the same with the barbell or dumbbells.

Stand up and assume a well-balanced position with your feet shoulder-width apart and your toes pointed straight ahead. Your arms should hang down but be inclined slightly forward so the weights will not touch your body. Secure the weights in the middle of the Strength Bar and hold the bar at the ends with a pronated grip. Keep your spine erect in its normal anatomical position (see Photo 7.1).

When you are ready, inhale slightly more than usual and then hold your breath as you raise your arms up and forward. Your arms should

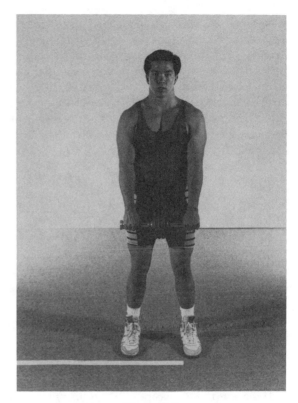

Photo 7.1

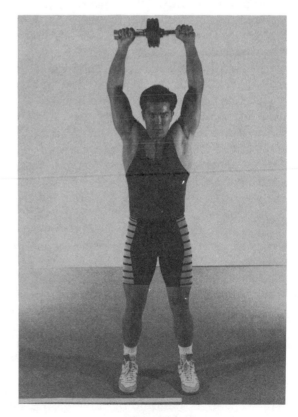

Photo 7.2

rise at least 45 degrees above the level of your shoulders or higher (see Photo 7.2). As you raise the weights, keep your trunk in the same position throughout the movement. Your arms should be kept straight or slightly bent if you feel any discomfort in the elbow joint. Upon reaching the uppermost position, relax somewhat and exhale as you return under control to the starting position.

Comments

- Heavy weights are not recommended, nor are they needed for proper and effective execution of this exercise. Because of the long lever created by your straight arms, a small weight seems to be very heavy when you hold it in your hands away from your body. Usually up to 20 pounds will challenge the strongest men when the exercise is done with strict form. Moreover, people who use very heavy weights have a tendency to hyperextend or arch their spine in order to raise the weight sufficiently high. This, in turn, produces great stress on the spine. Because the movement is usually vigorous, it can create excessive forces that can cause injury to the vertebrae and discs. Thus, you should use relatively light weights, not only for maximum effectiveness, but also for safety.
- The front arm raise exercise is also beneficial in increasing shoulder joint flexibility if you perform the exercise by raising your arms until they are directly overhead. In this way not only will you be developing flexibility, but you will also be gaining strength through the range of motion. This version of the exercise is also effective for improving posture. When you raise your arms overhead, you feel your rib cage lifting and your shoulders pulled to the rear.
- Most bodybuilders have a tendency to do this exercise with their elbows greatly bent so that they can handle greater weights. However, in so doing they move their elbows out to the sides so that, in essence, they are doing a partial lateral arm raise along with the front arm raise. Thus, if you must bend your elbows somewhat, be sure your upper arms are pointing forward so that the weights are in line with the midline of your body. To do this you have to use a narrower grip on the Strength Bar or regular barbell. However, such positioning is more stressful to the muscles. Thus, using lighter weights and going through the greater range is more productive.

- An effective variant of the front arm raise, especially for athletes, is the alternate dumbbell raise. In this exercise you work one arm at a time, which allows you to duplicate more closely the exact actions used in your sport. Also, when using dumbbells you can vary the pathway of the arm going up to make it a more natural movement. However, if you are looking for maximum anterior deltoid development, then you should do the exercise exactly the same as described with the Strength Bar.

■ Lateral Arm Raise on an Exercise Machine

Because the deltoids are so important in performance, safety, and appearance, there are many exercise machines that duplicate the lateral arm raise exercise. However, to get most effective development of the muscles when using a machine, it is important to do the exercise correctly.

With improper positioning, the exercise can be very dangerous to the shoulder joint. The exercise is described as performed on a Keiser lateral shoulder machine, which has the necessary adjustability and controls to allow you to do the exercise safely and in various ways.

Major muscles and actions involved

Lateral arm raises involve the deltoid and supraspinatus in shoulder joint abduction, when the arms are raised sideways from a position alongside the body (see Figure 7.11). The serratus anterior and the upper and lower trapezius are involved in upward rotation of the scapula, which accompanies the arm movement. In this action the scapulae rotate as follows: clockwise on the left side and counterclockwise on the right side when viewed from the rear.

Sports uses

The muscles used in raising your arms sideways (abduction) are most important in weightlifting and other iron sports. They are especially needed in exercises such as the top-pull in weightlifting (snatch and clean and jerk) and to a limited extent in powerlifting (deadlift). In bodybuilding and in general fitness, lateral raises are especially valuable. Because they develop the deltoid muscle, they produce the contour of the

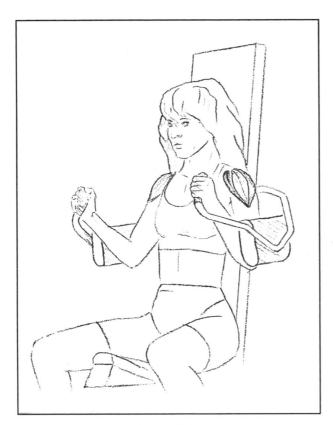

Figure 7.11
Muscles used in the lateral arm raise

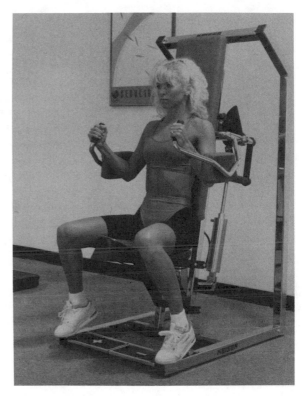

Photo 7.3

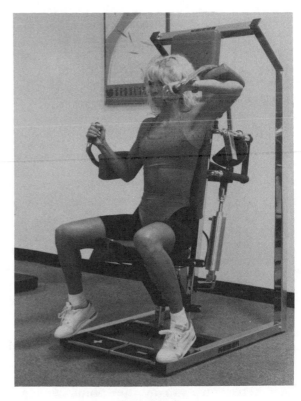

Photo 7.4

outside of the shoulders, give width to the shoulders, and give the body a V shape.

Shoulder joint abduction is a very important action in all sports that require athletes to raise their arms or reach up. Examples are blocking in basketball and volleyball, gymnastics (free exercise), diving takeoffs, catching overhead flies in baseball and passes in football, and the guarding stance and rebounding in basketball. (These movements are not done against a heavy resistance, however.) Also, bringing the arms overhead is used in football tackles; in the swimming dive, starting push-off, and recovery; and when raising the arm overhead to hit (the tennis serve, for example) or to throw (baseball, football, and so on).

One of the greatest values of doing lateral raises and developing the supraspinatus muscle is in providing safety and preventing injury. The supraspinatus is the main muscle holding the humerus in the glenoid fossa (the top of the shoulder joint), and it prevents shoulder joint dislocations.

Execution

Execution on the Keiser lateral shoulder raise machine will be described. Execution is basically the same on other machines. Adjust the seat height so that the axis of rotation in the machine lines up with the axis of rotation in your shoulder joints. When you are seated, grasp the handles and place your upper arms against the resistance lever pads (see Photo 7.3). Adjust the resistance with your finger, and then when you are ready, inhale and hold your breath. At the same time, raise both your arms sideways until they are 45 degrees or more above the horizontal. After reaching the uppermost position, exhale and return to the beginning position.

When using the Keiser machine you can also exercise each arm separately (see Photo 7.4). In this version you can achieve a slightly greater range of motion than when you work both arms at the same time.

Comments

• When you do the exercise unilaterally, you can have a decreased amount of resistance without having to make any adjustments on the machine. However, if you have narrow shoulders, you must slide your trunk over slightly to one side so that your shoulder axis lines up better with the axis of the machine. In this case, doing the exercise unilaterally rather than trying to do both arms at the same time can be safer for your shoulders. The reason for this is that if your shoulders are narrow, the resistance is located far from your shoulder joint, and thereby greater stress is placed on the shoulder joint.

• The Keiser machine can be used very effectively to change the resistance at different points in the range of motion. Because the exercise is difficult at mid-range if the resistance is great at the beginning, i.e., when your arms are alongside your body, you can decrease the resistance as you approach the horizontal so that you can go beyond it. Or, you can adjust the resistance when your arms are at approximately 45 degrees to the vertical and then go straight through the horizontal position to 45 degrees above it. In this way you work the deltoid through its most forceful range of motion. In addition, you can hold the horizontal position with greater resistance to develop the isometric strength at this point, which also helps to get beyond the sticking point.

• Lateral arm raises, when done through a full range of motion so that your arms are overhead, are also very important for full development of the upper and lower portions of the trapezius. This action is very important for developing the diamond shape in the middle of the back. There will also be maximum development of the deltoid muscle as it is worked through its entire range of motion. In the act of raising your arms completely overhead, the scapulae become elevated, which involves the very uppermost portion of the trapezius as well as the levator scapulae. This is the same action that occurs in the shrug exercise. Raising your arms completely overhead also maximally works the serratus anterior muscle, which plays a role in many different movements.

■ Lateral Dumbbell Arm Raise

This exercise is basically the same as the machine version. However, because the lateral dumbbell arm raise is so popular, its execution is also described. Note that the lever arm is much longer here so less resistance should be used.

Major muscles and actions involved

These are the same as in the machine lateral arm raise (see Figure 7.12).

Sports uses

The same as for the machine version.

Execution

Stand up and assume a well-balanced position with your feet shoulder-width apart and your toes pointed ahead or slightly to the sides. Hold a dumbbell in each hand with a neutral grip (with the ends of the dumbbell pointing forward and backward) and let your arms hang at your sides (see Photo 7.5). When you are ready, inhale slightly more than usual and then hold your breath as you raise your arms up and sideways, making sure to keep them straight, until they are at least 45 degrees above the horizontal or higher (see Photo 7.6). Your trunk should be maintained in the normal upright position throughout the movement. After reaching the uppermost position, relax your muscles slightly and exhale as you return the weights under control back to the original position.

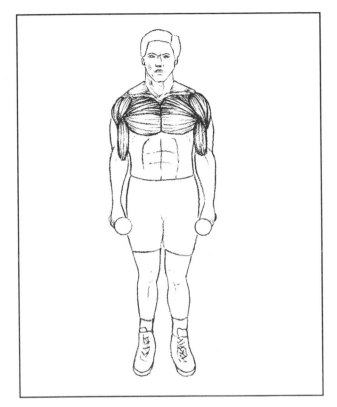

Figure 7.12
Muscles used in the lateral dumbbell arm raise

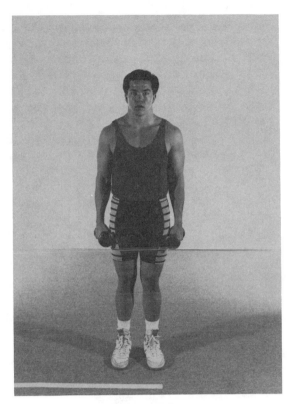

Photo 7.5

Comments

- When the lateral arm raise exercise is performed as described, major stress (resistance) is placed on the middle deltoid. To place greater resistance on the anterior portion of the deltoid, rotate your arms outwardly during the lift. To place greater stress on the posterior portion of the deltoid, rotate your arms inwardly during the lift.

- For variety, round your shoulders and drop your head down in the initial position. The dumbbells will then rest across the front of your thighs. Then, as you raise the dumbbells (they can also be swung), also raise your chest, head, and shoulders. These additional actions exercise the upper middle back muscles. In essence, they allow for development of the muscles that span the entire upper back. This is a vigorous motion, however, so be certain to hold your lower spine firm.

- For maximum effectiveness, extra heavy weights should not be used. Twenty to thirty pounds is usually plenty for most athletes and

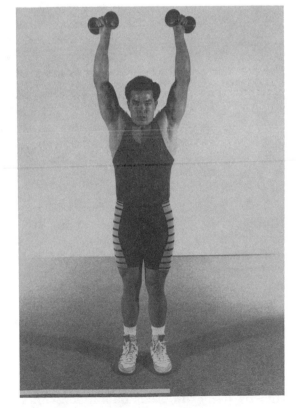

Photo 7.6

bodybuilders. Using great weight will change the biomechanics of the exercise (although this will not happen with machines such as the Keiser). For example, you will have to flex your elbows (which changes your elbow position) and you will not be able to raise the weights above the horizontal position. These changes in technique will not work the deltoid through its most favorable zone for development (45 degrees above and below the horizontal). Also, using extra heavy weights will eliminate some of the assisting muscles that are involved in this exercise. For example, the upper (clavicular) portion of the pectoralis major (which is involved only when the arm is above the horizontal) is eliminated, and the effect of the long head of the biceps brachii muscle is lessened when the elbow is flexed. Also very important is the fact that using lighter weights is less stressful to the body. This also applies to machine exercises.

• Keeping your arms relatively straight and going through a full range of motion with them is also very important for developing increased flexibility. If you do lateral arm raises and bring your arms to only a horizontal position, your shoulder joint will eventually tighten and it will become very difficult, if not impossible, to keep your arms straight and raise them completely above your head. However, raising your arms above your head is critical for effective performance of various sports and occupations.

Lat Pulldown

The lat pulldown is a very effective exercise that is used mainly for developing the upper latissimus dorsi to create "wings." The typical lat pulldown exercise has traditionally utilized a wide pronated grip. Today, however, many bodybuilders use a narrow grip, and when the exercise is done in this manner, different portions of the latissimus are used together with other secondary muscles. So, for full development of the latissimus and for different stress on the other major muscles, it is important that you do both wide grip and narrow grip variants. You can do this by using different bar attachments or by using a lat pulldown machine, such as the one

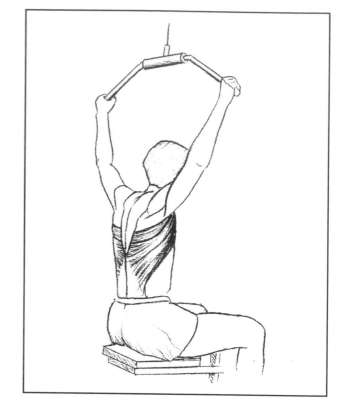

Figure 7.13
Muscles used in the lat pulldown

by Keiser on which you can execute both variants.

Major muscles and actions involved

In the pronated wide grip variant, the upper latissimus dorsi, the teres major, and the lower pectoralis major muscles are involved in shoulder joint adduction (see Figure 7.13). In this action your arms are pulled down in a side plane until your upper arm is below shoulder level. In the shoulder girdle, downward rotation of the scapulae is performed by the rhomboid and pectoralis minor muscles. In this action the right scapula rotates clockwise and the left counterclockwise (when viewed from the rear).

In the narrow neutral grip variant, the lower latissimus dorsi, the lower pectoralis major, and the teres major are involved in shoulder joint extension. In this action the arms move from in front of the body down to the sides of the trunk. This action is perpendicular to the lateral plane of the movement as in the wide grip variant. In the shoulder girdle the rhomboid, the pectoralis minor, and the middle trapezius are the major muscles involved in downward rotation and adduction of the scapulae. In this action the muscles pull the scapulae in toward the spine and at the same time rotate the right scapula clockwise and the left counterclockwise (when viewed from the rear).

Sports uses

The act of pulling your arms down from above your head or from in front of you sideways (or raising your body when your hands are secured as, for example, in climbing and pullups) is extremely important in many sports. For example, the action of shoulder joint adduction and/or extension is very important in the execution of stunts on the rings, horizontal bar, and uneven bars in gymnastics.

The muscles and actions are also important in pulling down rebounds in basketball, hand balancing (tandem), and in all pulling-up actions (climbing a ladder or wall and rock climbing). They arc also important for many holds in wrestling, for various phases of the pulling-pushing actions used in different swimming strokes, and in rowing, especially when the elbows are down.

Because the latissimus dorsi, and especially the teres major, are medial rotators in the shoulder joint, development of these muscles is important for pitchers and other athletes who must throw. These muscles are also needed in executing various downward blows as in breaking boards in karate and in other chopping actions.

For bodybuilders, this exercise is most important for development of the muscles noted, especially the latissimus dorsi. Full development of this muscle gives a broad appearance to the sides of the upper back and the lower back. It is also an important exercise for all athletes to help in maintaining a strong shoulder joint.

Execution

Execution on the Keiser machine will be described. If you use a different machine, you may have to change bars or make other adjustments to duplicate both variants.

For the pronated wide grip variant, adjust the height of the seat and sit down under the bar of a lat pulldown machine. The height of the seat must allow you to grasp the bar with your hands outstretched. When you are seated, place the padded leg bar over your thighs. Take a wide grip (hold the outermost ends) so that your arms form a wide V. Hold your arms in a fully extended position with your trunk and midsection straight and in line with your arms (see Photo 7.7).

Adjust the resistance with a press of your foot, and when you are ready, inhale and hold your breath as you pull down. Concentrate on bringing your elbows down and keeping your trunk in place. Flexion will occur in the elbow joints, but it should be a consequence of the adduction, that is, it should not be an active movement. Pull the bar down in back of your head until it is shoulder level or lightly touches the back of your neck or upper back (see Photo 7.8). Relax and exhale as you return the bar under control to the starting position and then repeat.

For the neutral narrow grip variant, assume the same position as in the wide grip variant. When you are properly seated, grasp the bar with the neutral grips, with your hands shoulder-width or slightly wider apart (see Photo 7.9).

When you are ready, inhale and hold your breath as you pull down at a moderate rate of speed. Concentrate on keeping your elbows down in front and your trunk erect. Flexion will occur in your elbow joints, but it should be mainly a consequence of the shoulder joint extension. Keep pulling down until the bar is chest high and your elbows are alongside your chest (see Photo 7.10). Relax slightly and exhale as you return the bar under control to the initial position.

Comments

- Because the entire latissimus dorsi is not involved in any one exercise, it is important that you do these two variants to develop the muscle fully. Development of the upper part of the latissimus dorsi will give you wings. Development of the lower part will give you great definition on the sides of your lower back. In addition, you will find that your sports performances improve greatly because of the more varied development. However, it is important to have an adjustable seat for proper positioning when you are grasping the bar. Also, the machine should have different grips to work the muscle completely.
- A machine such as the one by Keiser gives you the ability to regulate the resistance. Thus you can create a strong eccentric return, do isometric contractions at your sticking point, and increase or decrease the resistance by pressing a foot pedal. In this way you go through the full

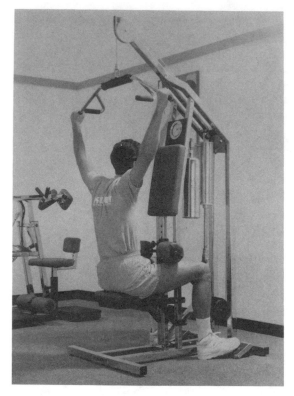

Photo 7.7

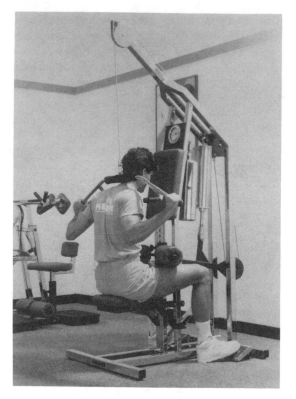

Photo 7.8

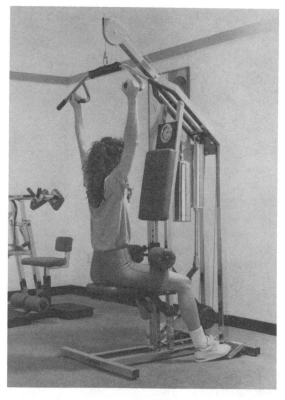

Photo 7.9

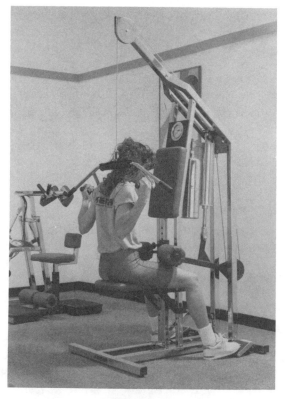

Photo 7.10

range of motion if you have trouble handling the weight that you chose.

- When you are using the wide grip, the exercise may feel easy in the upper range and difficult as the bar approaches your shoulders. If you experience this, it means that you are strong in the initial range of motion and weak in the bottom range. The Keiser machine is based on variable resistance that closely duplicates your strength curve. Therefore, when you use machines that do not have variable resistance, especially those with weight stacks, the exercise feels difficult in the early stages and even more so in the bottom position. To counteract this and to develop the muscle more effectively in the upper or lower range of motion, you can increase the resistance initially and work only the upper range. Or, as you are doing the exercise, you can have more resistance initially and then slowly decrease the resistance as you approach the bottom position where the exercise is more difficult. In this manner you can effectively work the entire range for full development of the muscle.

- When you use the narrow grip, it is important to keep your body erect so that you can more effectively work the lower lat in the upper range of motion. If you lean back, as many people do, you will be working only the lower range of motion. Thus, if you are looking for total development, it is a good idea to do both variants of the exercise with your trunk erect and also with your trunk inclined backward. However, when doing the exercise with your trunk inclined backward, it is important that you pull the bar down sufficiently so that your elbows go behind your body. You will notice that when you do this, the action is similar to that used in the seated row with a neutral grip.

- Using a seat with a padded bar that goes over your thighs to hold you down is very important for execution of the lat pulldown. If the bar to secure your body is not available, then you will find your body rising as you execute the pulldown when you use weights that are close to or greater than your body weight. Also, it is very important that the seat be adjusted so that your arms are maximally extended when you grab the bar. If you have to reach too high for the bar, it will be very difficult to keep your legs secured at the same time.

- An effective variant of the lat pulldown is the narrow grip pulldown, especially when done with a neutral grip. This version is analogous to the neutral grip pullup. In this exercise you get additional assistance from the posterior deltoid and the long head of the triceps. When you use the wide grip and shoulder adduction, the assisting muscles are the coracobrachialis, the subscapularis (when your arm is above the horizontal), the short head of the biceps, and the long head of the triceps.

- To execute the lat pulldown successfully, the scapulae must rotate downward as shoulder joint adduction takes place. If the shoulder girdle muscles are not strong enough to rotate the scapulae downward, the arms are not able to move down and the amount of shoulder adduction or extension is limited considerably. Also, there is a very good chance of injury to the muscles involved.

- An effective alternate exercise for the upper latissimus is the cable pulldown. To duplicate basically the same actions, however, be sure that you pull down the handles on a high pulley sideways toward the sides of your body. Pulling in front and crossing over changes the emphasis to the lower pectoral muscles in the lower range.

■ Seated Row

Many individuals use their back when they do the seated row on a low pulley and when they do the bent-over row. This not only limits the muscular involvement, but it also causes lower back problems, especially when the back is rounded. To prevent these problems and to do the exercise effectively, you should use an exercise machine such as the one made by Keiser that has both a neutral and a pronated grip. These two grips allow you to do the seated row in strict form and with some variety.

Major muscles and actions involved

Variant 1—*Neutral grip variant:* This variant includes shoulder joint extension, which involves the lower pectoralis major, the lower latissimus dorsi, and the teres major. The action is assisted by the posterior deltoid (see Figure 7.14). In this action your elbows move from a

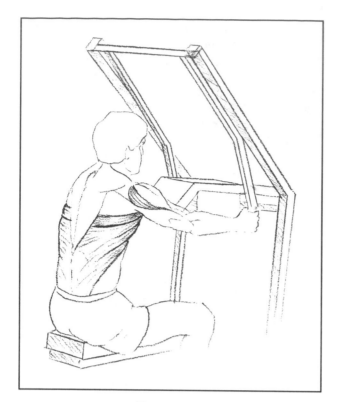

Figure 7.14
Muscles used in the seated row (neutral grip)

position in front of your body down and back until they are behind your trunk. Downward rotation and adduction of the scapulae occur in the shoulder girdle when your arms go beyond the level of your back. In this action the lower edges of the scapulae turn inward toward the spine while the upper edges of the scapulae are turned outward on an axis through the center of each scapula. As your arms go back past your body, both scapulae move in closer to one another and to the spine.

Variant 2—*Pronated grip variant:* In this variant the basic action is the same as the neutral grip variant because of the downward arc during execution. However, at the beginning, the posterior deltoid, the teres minor, and the infraspinatus are involved in shoulder joint horizontal extension. In this action your arms travel in a horizontal plane from a position in front of your body out to the sides and behind your trunk. In the shoulder girdle the middle trapezius and the rhomboid are involved in scapula adduction. In this action the scapulae move from an out-to-the-sides position on the rib cage to

close to the spine. In essence, they slide in toward one another and the spine. However, as you go through the full range of motion, the actions are basically the same as in the neutral grip variant.

Sports uses

Both variants of the seated row play an important role in all sports in which the arm is pulled to the rear. Thus they are important in the sports of rowing (sculls), gymnastics, tennis, racquetball, and badminton (executing backhands). Wrestlers also use this action when trying to keep their shoulders off the mat when getting pinned, and swimmers use shoulder extension in various strokes. Both variants are especially important in bodybuilding for development of the middle upper back, the posterior shoulder, and the lower sides of the back musculature.

Execution

Variant 1—*Neutral grip variant:* Adjust the seat of a seated row machine (the Keiser upper back machine) so that when you are in position your shoulders are level with the handles if they move horizontally backward. If the handles move downward in an arc, as in the Keiser machine (which is most effective for the neutral grip row) then you should position your shoulders slightly higher so that as the handles move backward and down, your elbows travel through a full range of motion. With the seat in position, adjust the chest plate so that when you grasp the neutral grips your arms will be fully extended and your shoulders slightly rounded. Your feet should be flat on the floor (or on the resistance levers with the Keiser machine) and your trunk erect to ensure proper action (see Photo 7.11).

When you are ready, inhale slightly more than usual and hold your breath as you pull the handles toward yourself. Keep your elbows down and moving back during the entire movement. In the end position, your elbows should be past the posterior surface of your shoulders, and your trunk should be in a slightly arched position (see Photo 7.12). After reaching the farthest position, relax your muscles somewhat and exhale as you return your arms to the original position under control. Pause momentarily and repeat in the same manner.

Variant 2—*Pronated grip variant:* Positioning in this variant is the same as with the neutral grip except that you use the pronated grip. To

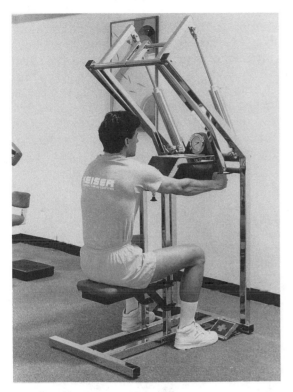

Photo 7.11

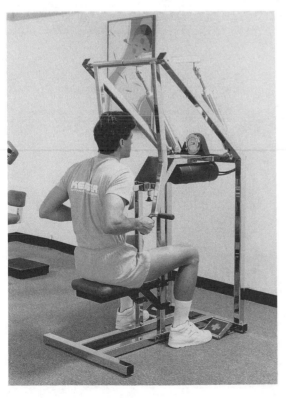

Photo 7.12

execute, inhale slightly more than usual and hold your breath as you pull back and down with your arms. Keep your elbows out to the sides and pull until they are past the level of the back of your trunk. However, because your elbows are also moving down, your hands finish up close to your stomach area. Exhale as you return to the initial position, keeping the movement under control.

Comments

- When using the pronated grip, it is important that you keep your elbows out to the sides as you execute the exercise. If you keep your elbows in close to your sides, instead of having some horizontal shoulder abduction and extension taking place, you will be doing only shoulder extension. In this case, the neutral grip is better suited for greater development. In addition, adduction of the scapulae (which occurs strongly in the pronated grip) is the only action of the middle trapezius. For maximum shortening, the elbows must be out to the sides and must go beyond the level of the back. If you are seeking strict form, you should also do lateral prone raises (described later in the chapter).

- To ensure proper technique and the resulting correct muscle involvement, your trunk must remain basically stationary and erect. Your trunk should have no backward lean to assist in pulling the handles to your chest. If this occurs, your lower back muscles (erector spinae) are doing the work, not your shoulder girdle and shoulder joint muscles. This is why you must keep your chest in contact with the chest pad at all times. The key to safe and effective execution is to keep your lower spine in its normal slightly arched position at all times. This is especially true if you use a freestanding T-bar or if you execute a bent-over row.

- There should not be any active elbow joint flexion with either grip. If you actively execute elbow joint flexion, you will not be using your shoulder joint and back muscles to the necessary extent. In essence, this prevents your elbows from going as far to the rear as possible, which limits the action of the muscles involved.

  Some active muscular contractions occur in the elbow joints as a consequence of the shoulder joint movement. These are needed to hold the elbow joint in place, not to forcefully execute elbow flexion. Concentration must be on the shoulder action.

■ Bent-Over Dumbbell Row

The bent-over dumbbell row with the neutral grip is a good substitute for the neutral grip seated row. To execute, bend over from your hips with your side to an exercise bench. Your back should be in its normal slightly arched position from your hips to your head. Flex your legs slightly at your knees for greater stability. Support your upper body with your free arm by resting it on the bench. Hold a dumbbell in your other hand and keep your shoulder rounded (protracted). See Photo 7.13.

When you are in position, inhale slightly more than usual and hold your breath as you pull the dumbbell up. Concentrate on raising your elbow as high as possible using your back muscles. Keep your trunk in a stable position during the pulling action. In the uppermost position your elbow should be above the level of your back and your shoulder should be raised (retracted) slightly (see Photo 7.14). Exhale as you lower the dumbbell to the straight-arm position under control. When you complete your repetitions with one arm, move to the other side of the bench and repeat the exercise with your other arm.

It is important that your body be kept stationary during execution of this exercise. To ensure this, shift most of your weight to the support arm to stabilize your body. Because of the extra support, this exercise is usually preferred to the freestanding bent-over or T-bar row. Also, because you use less weight, there is less stress on your spine, which makes this exercise safer. To duplicate the pronated grip seated row, hold

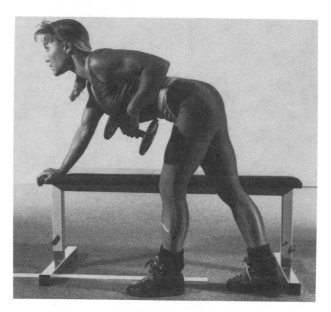

Photo 7.14

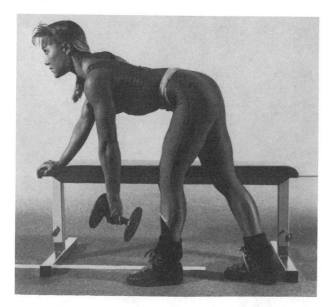

Photo 7.13

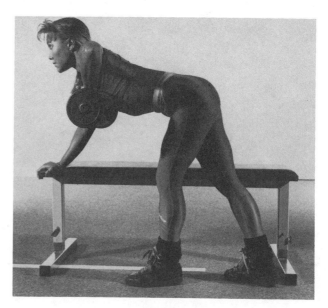

Photo 7.15

your elbow out to the side in line with your shoulders and execute in the same manner as the neutral grip variant (see Photo 7.15).

Lateral Prone Raise (Reverse Fly)

Most sports and occupations require working with the arms in front of the body. In time, this causes round shoulders and in some cases the appearance of a sunken chest. To counteract this tendency and to improve posture at the same time, the lateral prone raise in strict form, also known as the reverse fly, should be done.

Major muscles and actions involved

In the reverse fly the muscles of the shoulder joint are the middle and posterior deltoid, the infraspinatus, and the teres minor (see Figure 7.15). They are involved in horizontal extension (abduction) in which your arms are brought from a position in front of your body (hanging down vertically with the trunk horizontal) up and to your sides until they are in line with your shoulders and above the level of your back. In the shoulder girdle the rhomboid and the middle fibers of the trapezius are involved in scapula adduction. In this action the scapulae move from the sides of the chest to a position close to the spine.

Sports uses

Shoulder joint horizontal abduction and scapula adduction always take place when your arm is pulled to the rear in a horizontal plane (in relation to the body). This is used in the sports of rowing (sculls), gymnastics (iron cross on the rings), tennis, racquetball, and badminton (shoulder high backhand), baseball batting in the left shoulder of a right-handed batter (high pitch), and archery (the pull back). At times, wrestlers use this action when trying to keep their shoulders off the mat when they are pinned down. You will note that many of these uses also apply to the seated row.

Lateral prone raises are very important to bodybuilders for development of the middle upper back musculature and the upper and posterior surface of the shoulders.

Execution

Assume a prone position on a narrow exercise bench so that your entire trunk rests on the seat. Hold dumbbells in your hands in a neutral grip (palms toward each other) and let your arms hang straight down, perpendicular to your trunk (see Photo 7.16). In this position your shoulders should be slightly protracted (lower than the top of the bench). If you use a low bench, keep your

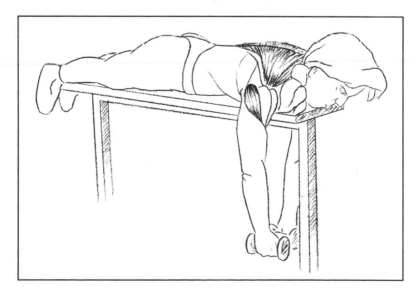

Figure 7.15
Muscles used in the lateral prone raise (reverse fly)

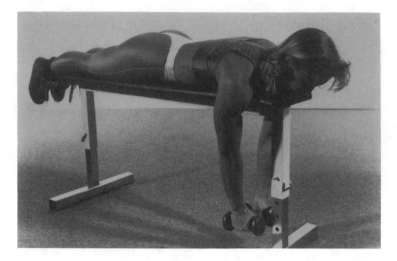

Photo 7.16

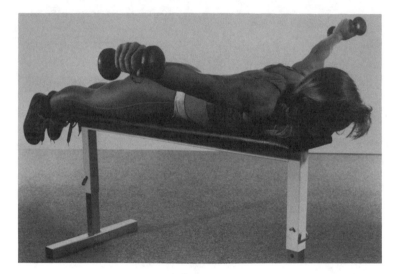

Photo 7.17

arms out to the sides with the dumbbells on the floor.

When you are ready, inhale slightly more than usual and hold your breath as you raise your arms sideways in line with your shoulders as high as possible. Do the movement fairly vigorously so that you are able to raise the weights high enough. In the ending position the weights and your elbows should be higher than your back (see Photo 7.17). After reaching the uppermost position, relax your muscles slightly and exhale as you lower the dumbbells under control to the initial position. Pause momentarily and repeat.

Comments

- In the shoulder girdle the lateral prone raise exercise involves the middle fibers of the trapezius maximally (as does the T-bar or bent-over row with the pronated grip, that is, elbows up and out to the sides). The reason for this is that scapula adduction is the only function of this portion of the trapezius muscle.

- The trapezius and rhomboid muscles are very important in making a full range of motion possible for the arms. By pulling the scapulae back toward the spine, the shoulder joint sockets are turned slightly backward. This allows

118

your upper arms to be raised level with and behind your back.

- Lateral prone raises become much more difficult when your arm is kept extended. In this position the weight is farther away from your body, which creates a longer resistance arm. Because of this, there is no need to use heavy weights, which would place more stress on the body and change the technique of execution.

The key element in the reverse fly is how high your elbow (arm) gets. The higher it is, the greater is the shortening contraction of the muscles involved. When you use heavy weights, however, you will have to bend your elbows, which changes the joint actions and the muscles involved. Flexing your elbows slightly is permissible, especially if you feel discomfort in the elbows. When you flex your elbows to a great extent, they drop so that the movement is done on a diagonal pathway, not perpendicular to the trunk.

- This exercise is most effective when executed on a high, narrow bench so that the dumbbells clear the floor in the starting position. This allows you to start with your arms straight and thus prevent excessive elbow joint flexion, which occurs when you use a low exercise bench and start with the weights under the seat. In addition, the high bench allows for a greater range of motion. In the starting position your shoulders will be protracted and your scapulae will be pulled away from the spine (abducted). This forces the muscles to work through a greater range under resistance to bring your shoulders back (middle trapezius and rhomboid) in order to raise the weights much higher than your back. This is similar to what occurs on the Keiser machine.

- This exercise is safer and more effective for isolation of the muscles involved than the bent-over row and the T-bar row. It is very difficult to hold your spine in an arched position when doing the bent-over row, and, in addition, there is a strong tendency to use your trunk when pulling upward, and this can be dangerous. Therefore, when using a T-bar, use one with a chest support to eliminate use of your trunk. Most T-bars are effective for use with the neutral grip, but because of the angle of incline when you use the pronated grip, it is impossible to move your arms perpendicular to your trunk. Because of this, you cannot get

full development of the posterior deltoid, teres minor, and infraspinatus as is possible in the lateral prone raise.

■ Seated Butterfly

When it comes to doing the fly, the machine exercise is often preferred because it allows for strict form, especially when heavy weights are used. In addition, when you use machines such as the one by Keiser, you can get a multitude of muscular contractions to get the exact muscle development that you seek, that is, upper, lower, or the midsection of the pectoralis major.

Major muscles and actions involved

Horizontal adduction, which involves the anterior deltoid, coracobrachialis, and pectoralis major muscles, occurs in the shoulder joint (see Figure 7.16). In this action your arms move from an out-to-the-sides position toward the midline of your chest. Your arms remain on a level with your shoulders. In addition, the serratus anterior and pectoralis minor muscles are involved in shoulder girdle abduction. In this action the scapulae move away from the spine out toward the sides of the rib cage.

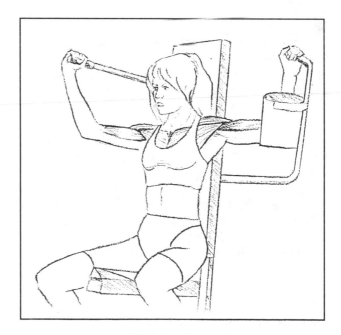

Figure 7.16
Muscles used in the seated butterfly

Sports uses

The combination of shoulder joint horizontal flexion and shoulder girdle abduction is very important in sports that require forward reaching and grabbing actions. These actions are used in the sports of gymnastics (rings, parallel bars, free exercises), boxing (round house), martial arts (execution of various punches), football (tackling and grabbing an opponent from the side), and in powerlifting (bench press). In bodybuilding this exercise is very important for chest and anterior shoulder muscle development. In addition, the exercise also aids development of the muscles in the area under the armpits (serratus anterior).

Execution

The following description is based on the use of an exercise machine, more specifically, the one made by Keiser. Before beginning, adjust the seat of the machine so that when you are in a seated position your upper arms are perpendicular to your trunk when you place your forearms against the resistance lever pads in front of you. Your feet should be placed so that they are able to make contact with the controls to adjust the amount of resistance, which should be zero at this time. Your trunk should rest against the back support as you place your forearms in a vertical or slightly angled position against the resistance arm pads in front of you (see Photo 7.18).

When you are in position with your arms in front of you, increase the resistance as needed and prepare yourself for execution. Inhale slightly more than usual and hold your breath as you bring your arms to the rear (see Photo 7.19) through the necessary range of motion and then return them to the front. Exhale as you approach the front position, in which both your elbows should be facing forward. Generally speaking, a full range of motion can be attained when the elbows go slightly past the line of the shoulders. When you have completed the necessary number of repetitions, decrease the resistance before releasing the forearm pads to return them to the rear position.

Comments

• Breathing rhythm is very important in the execution of this exercise. When you inhale, your rib cage (chest) expands and stabilizes so

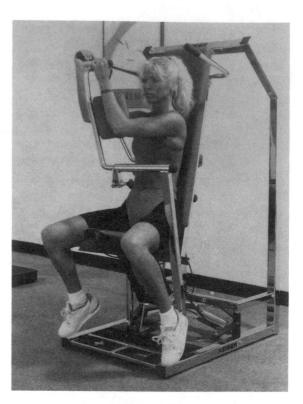

Photo 7.18

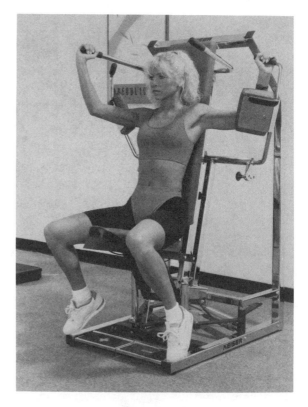

Photo 7.19

that the muscles have a firm base upon which to pull during their contraction. If your rib cage is not held firm, your ribs will move as your muscles contract, resulting in less force and the potential for greater stress, especially on the backward movement.

- The movement should be under control at all times. You should not relax your muscles in the most backward position unless you use light resistance and are looking for increased flexibility. When the resistance is great, you should quickly reverse directions once your arms have passed your back. Allowing the eccentric return to bring your arms all the way to the rear with your muscles relaxed can cause tearing of the pectoralis or anterior deltoid. This is especially true when doing the dumbbell fly.

- The butterfly exercise is one of the best exercises to fully develop the middle of the pectoralis major muscle. This is the only exercise in which both the upper and lower muscle fibers are involved; all other actions which involve the pectorals use only the upper or lower portions. To ensure that the entire pectoralis is worked, you must keep your arms perpendicular to your trunk when executing this exercise. Note that doing this exercise with dumbbells is difficult unless you use light weights and keep your arms straight. If very heavy weights are used, you will have to bend your elbows to accommodate the extra weight, which tends to make you drop your elbows so that the weight stays in line with your shoulders. If you drop your elbows, you will be working more of the lower pectoralis major and therefore not including the upper portion.

- If you wish to work the lower pectorals on an exercise machine, adjust the seat higher so that when you exercise, your elbow will be pointed down approximately 10–20 degrees. If you desire more upper development, drop the seat very slightly so that your elbow is in line with or is slightly higher than your upper shoulders.

- The Keiser machine also gives you the option of using one arm alone. The exercise performed in this manner is very effective for developing greater flexibility in the shoulder joint and shoulder girdle. To execute, allow your shoulder girdle to go into retraction on the return, and, when your arms move for-

ward, into protraction. In this way you gain a greater range of motion and more closely duplicate most sports movements.

In addition, with the Keiser machine this exercise can be done at a high speed. However, to do so, you must decrease the range of motion and reverse positions when your elbow is in line with your shoulders or just slightly to the rear. When doing fast repetitions, however, do not use great resistance because the stress can be quite great on the shoulder joint.

- When using other butterfly machines (also known as "pec decks"), be careful not to overstretch your arms in the rear position because the stress in this range can be severe. When you use the Keiser machine, you decrease the resistance so that you can move the pads into position without any resistance. With other machines, you must set the resistance before assuming your seated position.

Another very effective exercise is the cable crossover, but only if you do it while you are lying on your back between two low cables. The key here is to use a relatively light weight and to keep your arms straight so that the weight can travel in a perpendicular direction to your trunk. In essence, this is exactly the same as doing the dumbbell fly. However, if you use heavy weights you will have to bend your elbows, and when this happens, you will be working the lower pectorals but not the upper.

■ Upright Row

There are only a few exercises that maximally work the middle head of the deltoid muscle. One of the better ones is the upright row, but only if it is done correctly. Doing it incorrectly can cause your shoulders to slope.

Major muscles and actions involved

In the shoulder joint the middle deltoid and supraspinatus are involved in shoulder abduction. In this action the upper arms move from a position alongside and slightly in front of the body out to the sides until they are above the level of the shoulders. The middle deltoid and supraspinatus are assisted in this action by the anterior and posterior deltoid, the clavicular portion of the pectoralis major (when the arm is

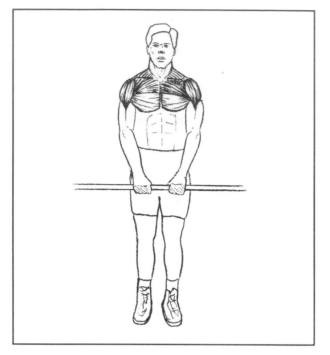

Figure 7.17
Muscles used in the upright row

Execution

Stand up with your feet approximately shoulder-width apart. Using a pronated grip, hold a barbell in your hands with your hands about eight inches apart. Extend your arms fully so that the barbell rests across your upper thighs (see Photo 7.20). When you are in position, take a slightly greater than normal breath and hold it as you lift the barbell straight up. As you pull, concentrate on pulling with your deltoid and upper back muscles so that the action is concentrated in your shoulder joints. Keep your hands as close to your body as possible while keeping your elbows out and back. Also, keep your body erect during the entire pull. In the finish position your elbows should be up and pointing out at approximately a 30–40 degree angle above the horizontal (see Photo 7.21).

After reaching the uppermost position, relax your muscles slightly and lower the barbell slowly so that it is under control at all times. Exhale on the return and repeat.

Comments

- In order to get full development of the middle head of the deltoid, it is critical that you keep the barbell close to you with your elbows out to the sides and back. In essence, you want your upper arm to be in the same plane as your shoulders at all times. If you let your elbows wander to a position in front of your body, even for a few degrees, the stress will switch to the anterior deltoid. This will negate the main purpose of this exercise.
- It is also important to maintain an upright position throughout the entire execution. Your spine should be in its normal anatomical position so that you maintain a slight arch in your lower back. If you relax your spine or lean forward slightly, it will be more difficult to raise the barbell to maximum height. Also, there will be a tendency for the barbell to move away from your body—and when this happens you will be stressing the anterior and not the middle deltoid. You may also be placing unwanted stress on the inner portions of the spinal discs, which, in time, can be dangerous. Holding your breath assists greatly in maintaining an upright position and a firm spine.
- To ensure proper execution of the upright row, you must not use excessively heavy weights. Doing so will limit the range of motion greatly and you will not get maximum development of

above the horizontal), and the long head of the biceps brachii (see Figure 7.17).

In the shoulder girdle the upper and lower portions of the trapezius and the serratus anterior rotate the scapulae upward. In this action the right scapula rotates counterclockwise and the left scapula rotates clockwise when viewed from the rear. Because the shoulder girdle is elevated, the levator scapulae is also involved (together with the uppermost trapezius). In this action the scapulae move upward in a vertical line.

Sports uses

The actions involved in the upright row are used in all sports that require lifting or pulling actions. This includes football (raising the arms to block or tackle), weightlifting (the top pull before the squat under), and gymnastics (inverted pulls on the rings, high bar, and parallel bars). The greatest value of the upright row is in development of the muscles of the upper and lower middle back and shoulders. Not only is this exercise very effective for producing muscle definition, but it also helps to develop wider, more level shoulders.

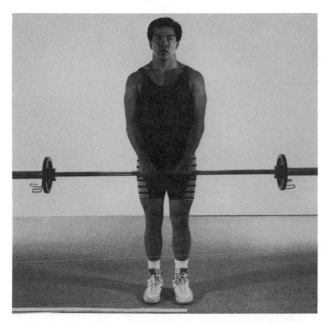

Photo 7.20

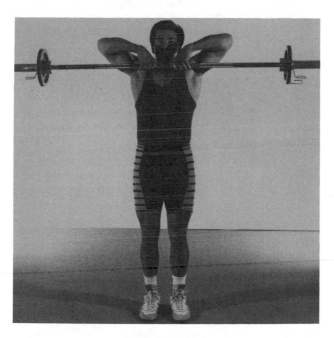

Photo 7.21

- By raising your elbows up as high as possible, you also get greater involvement of the upper and lower trapezius. When this muscle is well developed, it appears as a diamond shape in the middle of the upper back. In addition, in the upright row you get greater serratus anterior involvement in maximum range motion. Thus you can get excellent development of three muscles from doing just one exercise.
- It is important to do this exercise with a narrow grip in order to ensure a maximum range of motion. When you assume a wide grip, you will not be able to raise your elbows high enough. However, if your grip is *too* narrow (hands together), your elbows will have to move forward, you will not be able to get the bar high enough, and you will find it more difficult to balance the bar.
- For variety and even greater involvement of other muscles, you can do the continuous pull exercise. In this exercise you begin in the normal bent-leg deadlift position with your back in its normal, slightly arched position and your arms fully extended holding the barbell. Then execute the deadlift until you get to almost the final position and then begin the upright row without any stopping of the barbell movement. You may notice that movement is easier in the initial stages of the upright row, and this is fine because the major work of the muscles is done when your elbows are at a 45-degree angle above the horizontal. By doing two exercises in one, you develop greater coordination, which is most useful for athletes and also is of great benefit to bodybuilders.
- It should be noted that elbow flexion also occurs. In this action the elbow flexors (biceps brachii, brachialis, and brachioradialis) also undergo contraction, but the movement is passive. These muscles do not lift the bar. The shoulder joint action raises the bar and the elbow flexors contract to hold the elbow joint and bar in place.

the muscles. It is important to understand that the deltoid muscle is most active in the middle range of the total range of motion possible in the shoulder joint. It does most of its work from approximately 45 degrees below the horizontal to 45 degrees above the horizontal. For athletes, full-range motion is critical for protection from dislocations.

■ Pullover

The pullover is an exercise that not only develops the muscles but also increases the size of the chest. It is commonly executed with your arms bent or held straight.

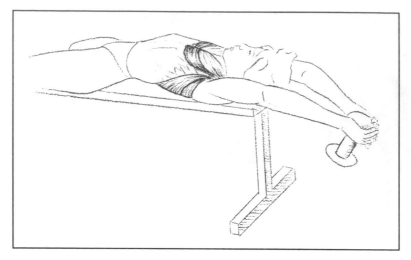

Figure 7.18
Muscles used in the pullover

Major muscles and actions involved

In the shoulder joint extension occurs, which involves the pectoralis major (lower portion), latissimus dorsi (lower portion), and teres major (see Figure 7.18). In this action the arms are raised upward from a horizontal position over the head (the body is also horizontal). In the shoulder girdle the rhomboid and pectoralis minor are the major muscles involved in downward rotation of the scapulae. In this action the right scapula rotates clockwise and the left counterclockwise when viewed from the rear.

Sports uses

The act of pulling your arms from an overhead position toward your body (or raising your body with your arms when your hands are secured in one place, as in chinning) is extremely important in gymnastics (rings, horizontal bar, uneven bars, and parallel bars). In addition, the movement used in the pullover is very important in all overhead forward throwing actions involving both arms (basketball, soccer throw-ins, medicine ball throwing), pulling down rebounds in basketball, the hit and follow-through phase in high volleyball spiking, hand balancing (tandem), and in all pulling-up actions (rope climbing, pullups). Wrestlers need this movement in many holds and swimmers require this very important action in various phases of the pulling phase in different strokes. For bodybuilders this exercise is very important for development of the

muscles noted, for increasing the size of the chest by expanding the rib cage, and for improving breathing capabilities.

Execution

Lie face up (supine) on an exercise bench so that you are well balanced with your trunk and pelvic girdle on the bench and your feet on the floor. Your body should be positioned so that your elbows clear the end of the bench when your upper arms are overhead (back). With your arms straight, hold a dumbbell above your chest. Be sure to hold the inner plate of the dumbbell so that the shaft remains vertical throughout the movement, and keep your arms straight or slightly flexed at the elbows at all times. Bring the dumbbell over your head and down until your upper arms are in line with your trunk. A slightly lower position can be attained if you have the needed shoulder joint flexibility (see Photo 7.22). As you lower the weight, take a deep breath to greatly expand your rib cage. When you reach the lowermost position, hold your breath. Then, raise the dumbbell up until it is directly above your chest (see Photo 7.23). Exhale after you pass the most difficult portion of the lift. Pause momentarily and then repeat.

Comments

• In order to get maximum benefit from the pullover exercise, you must concentrate on pulling with your shoulder joint muscles, not your arm muscles. If you do the exercise with

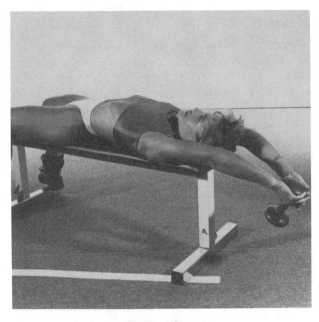

Photo 7.22   Photo 7.23

your elbows bent, which is very common among bodybuilders, you may find yourself doing elbow joint extension to raise the dumbbell.

• Individuals who use the bent-elbow technique do so in an effort to handle more weight. However, a light weight with your arms straight can create the same amount of tension in the muscle as a weight two to three times as heavy but with your arms bent. Also, when you bend your arms up to 90 degrees, you will have a tendency not to lower your elbows sufficiently to get maximum expansion of your rib cage, or even a full range of motion, and then you will not get some of the key benefits from this exercise.

• When you first start doing this exercise, it is important that you keep your lower spine in its natural, slightly arched position. Do not allow it to arch extensively, because this will unbalance the basic position and may lead to injury. Excessive arching usually occurs when you have insufficient flexibility in your shoulder joints. If this is the case, you should gradually work up to a full range of motion. Instead of trying to lower the dumbbell until your upper arms are horizontal, lower it to the point where the excessive arching begins and then stop and hold while your muscles relax.

This will stretch the muscles and connective tissue.

• One of the great values of the pullover is that it aids in breathing, and also in the expansion of the chest cage. Because of this, it is important that you take a deep breath as you lower your arms. This results in a stretching of the muscles that lift and expand the rib cage, and a contraction of these muscles during the exhalation phase.

■ Shoulder Shrug

The shoulder shrug is typically done with free weights. However, because heavy weights are usually used, tremendous stress is placed on the spine and shoulders, especially in the resting position. To counteract this tendency, you can do the exercise on an exercise machine such as the one made by Keiser.

Major muscles and actions involved

In the shrug there is elevation of the clavicle and scapula, which involves the upper trapezius, levator scapulae, and rhomboids (see Figure

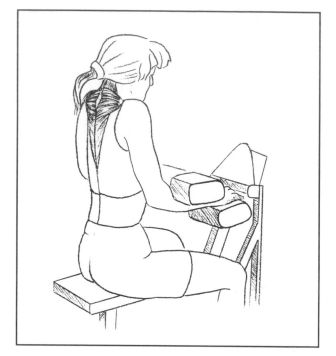

Figure 7.19
Muscles used in the shoulder shrug

Execution

Because of its greater safety and ease of execution, shrugs on the Keiser shrug machine will be described. However, execution with free weights is basically the same except for the placement of your hands. Adjust the seat so that when you are in an erect seated position with your feet on the floor close to the air resistance pedals, there is some tension on your forearms and your shoulders are sloped downward. Decrease the resistance completely, bend your trunk, and place your forearms between the resistance lever bars with your palms down. Then straighten your trunk to the erect position with your elbows at a 90-degree angle (see Photo 7.24). Increase the resistance and prepare for the shrug.

When you are ready, inhale and hold your breath as you pull your shoulders up as high as possible. As you elevate your shoulders, keep your arms vertical and your shoulders back. Continue this movement until your neck becomes hidden between your shoulders (see Photo 7.25). After reaching the uppermost position, exhale and lower your shoulders to a downward sloped position. Keep the movement under control at all times and your eyes focused straight ahead.

Comments

- It is interesting to note the action of the uppermost fibers of the trapezius muscles. When your head is free to move (not held firmly in place), contraction of the trapezius muscles on both sides of your head will tilt your head backward, raising your chin. If this happens, you will not be able to raise your shoulders. Therefore, to ensure that you do the exercise effectively, you must keep your head in place with your eyes focused directly in front of you. Doing this will also prevent you from leaning backward during execution, an action which can place excessive pressure on your spine.
- The muscles involved in this exercise are very powerful, and because of this you can overcome a great resistance. However, be sure that the resistance you are handling does not limit your range of motion. It is very important that you raise your shoulders as high as you can and basically hide your neck. When the resistance is very great or the seat is too high, your shoulders will be forced down too far at the beginning of the exercise, making it impossible for you to raise them above the horizontal.

7.19). In this action the shoulder girdle is raised upward (vertically).

Sports uses

Shoulder elevation is needed in all sports that require the shoulders for getting maximum reach. Thus it is important in football blocking and tackling and in executing weightlifting cleans. It is also important in reaching as high as possible to catch a ball as in baseball or football; and hitting a ball from the highest position, such as in the volleyball spike, tennis overhead, and tennis serve. For the horizontal bar exercises in gymnastics, shoulder elevation (and depression) is the key action needed to elongate the body to slow it down after it has been swinging. (In depression the body's radius is shortened.)

The shrug is especially important to bodybuilders and football players for development of the muscles on both sides of the neck and the inner shoulders. No other exercise develops the muscles through as great a range of motion with as much muscle isolation. It should also be noted that shoulder elevation is necessary to keep the shoulders from sloping when heavy objects are carried in the hands.

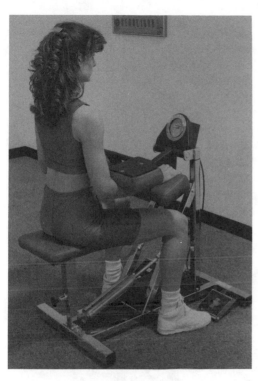

Photo 7.24

Doing this for a prolonged period of time will bulk up the trapezius, but it will develop in an elongated state and will not be capable of holding the shoulders up to give you square shoulders.

- It is also important that you keep your shoulders back as much as possible when you do this exercise. With the barbell this becomes fairly difficult, but with the machine or dumbbells there should be no problem. By keeping your shoulders back you maintain good posture and develop the muscles in a manner that will keep your shoulders in a good posture position.

- An effective variant of this exercise is the shoulder circle with dumbbells. To execute this version, begin with your shoulders rounded and sloping, then raise your shoulders up as high as possible, then back as far as possible, then down, and then forward and up again. In this version you also do protraction and retraction of the shoulder girdle.

- The Keiser machine is also well suited for developing strength at any specific point in the

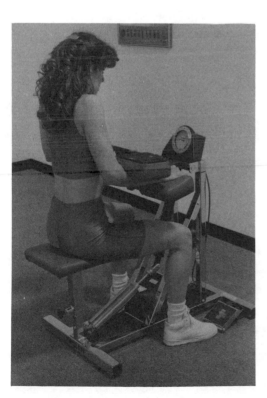

Photo 7.25

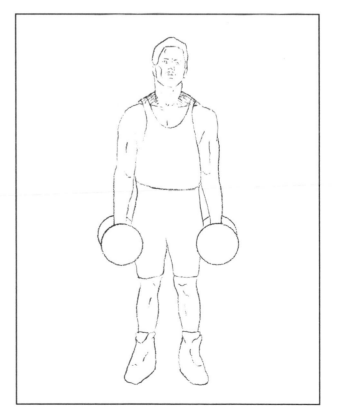

Figure 7.20
Muscles used in the shoulder shrug with dumbbells

range of motion. By increasing or decreasing the resistance with the press of your foot, you can regulate the exact amount of resistance needed. In this way you can go through the entire range of motion with maximum resistance. Or, if you are an athlete, you can do the exercise quickly, but if you do so, be sure that you pull with your shoulders and not with your arms.

- If a machine is not available, you can do shoulder shrugs in the same manner with free weights (see Figure 7.20). To do so, stand erect and hold a dumbbell in each hand (see Photo 7.26). When you are ready, inhale and hold your breath as you raise your shoulders as high as possible (see Photo 7.27). Return to the initial position, exhale, and repeat.

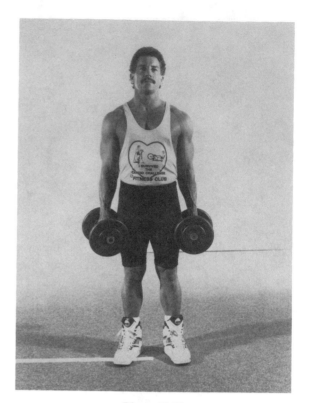

Photo 7.26

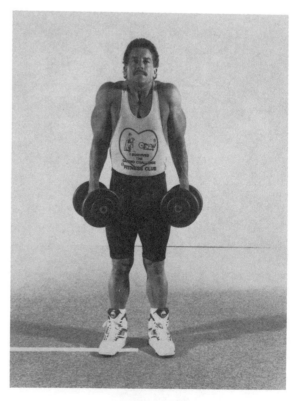

Photo 7.27

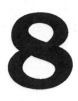 **The Elbow Joint**

ANATOMY OF THE ELBOW JOINT

The elbow joint is a hinge joint formed by the junction of the humerus and the radius and ulna bones of the lower arm. Strong ligaments hold the joint together in addition to the muscles and tendons. There is also movement between the radius and ulna bones, which allows for pronation and supination of the forearm.

BASIC MOVEMENTS IN THE ELBOW JOINT

In flexion the forearm moves toward the upper arm or vice versa. In extension the forearm moves away from the upper arm in an arm-straightening action. The reverse action, in which the upper arm moves away from the forearm, is also possible.

MAJOR MUSCLES INVOLVED

The major flexor muscles of the elbow joint are the biceps brachii, brachialis, and brachioradialis muscles (see Figures 8.1 and 8.2). The biceps brachii has a long and a short head. The division between them can be seen in bodybuilders in whom this muscle is well developed and who have little fat in the area. In the shoulder joint the long head of the biceps is attached to the scapula at the top of the glenoid cavity,

and the short head is attached to the coracoid of the scapula. At the lower end, the two heads blend into a common muscle and tendon which crosses the elbow joint and attaches to the tuberosity of the radius (close to the elbow joint).

The brachialis is located between the biceps and the humerus near the elbow. It originates on the anterior surface of the lower half of the humerus and inserts on the tuberosity of the ulna and the coronoid process of the ulna.

The brachioradialis is found on the outer surface of the forearm and creates the rounded contour from the elbow to the thumb. Its origin is on the upper two thirds of the lateral supracondyloid ridge of the humerus (close to the elbow) and insertion is on the lateral surface of the radius at the base of the styloid process (very close to the wrist).

It is interesting to note the differences and changes in strength of the various flexor muscles at different angles. For example, when the elbow is flexed 90 degrees, the brachialis is almost as strong as the biceps; the brachioradialis is about half as strong, and the pronator teres is about one-tenth as strong.

Only one major muscle is involved in elbow joint extension—the triceps brachii, which is a large muscle that covers the entire back side of the upper arm (see Figure 8.3). It is divided into three sections, known as the lateral (outer) head, medial (middle) head, and long (inner) head. The lateral head originates on the back of the humerus from the middle of the shaft to almost the very top. The medial head originates on the

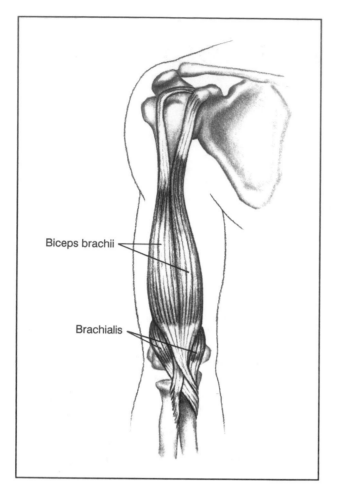

Figure 8.1
Anterior view of the upper right arm

ELBOW JOINT EXERCISES: BICEPS CURL VARIANTS

To describe the biceps curl and the myriad of ways in which it is executed requires a separate book. Because of the great variety of exercises, it is very difficult to isolate only a few that are most popular yet most effective. However, after carefully analyzing all the different exercises, I found that many of them are used to develop the elbow flexors in different ranges of motion. Because of this, I divided the exercises into three groups: those that are effective for development of muscles in the beginning straight-arm range of motion, those effective in the mid-range of motion with bent arms to the 90-degree angle or slightly above the 90-degree angle, and those that are maximally effective in the mid-range and beyond the 90-degree angle.

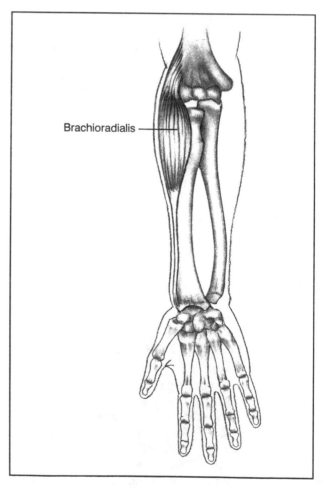

Figure 8.2
Anterior view of the lower right arm

lower portion of the back of the humerus over a wide space extending nearly two-thirds of the length of the bone. The long head of the triceps originates on the scapula just below the shoulder joint.

All three heads come together into a common tendon which inserts on the olecranon process of the ulna. It should be noted that the olecranon process extends beyond the elbow joint and prevents excessive hyperextension. To work all portions of the triceps muscle maximally, increasingly heavy weights must be used. For example, when light or moderately heavy weights are used, only the medial head of the triceps goes into action. As the resistance increases, the lateral head joins in, and when sufficiently heavy weights are used, the long head goes into contraction.

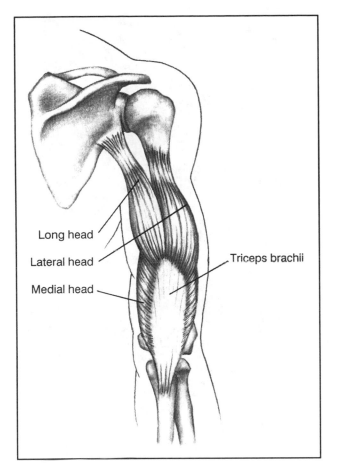

Figure 8.3
Posterior view of the upper right arm

Beginning Range Biceps Curl with a Barbell or Dumbbells

Major muscles and actions involved

In the biceps curl exercise, the biceps brachii, brachialis, and brachioradialis muscles are involved in elbow joint flexion (see Figure 8.4). In this action the forearm moves toward the upper arm from a fully extended position of the arm.

Sports uses

The greatest value of this biceps curl variant is in pulling (lifting) actions from a straight-arm position. These are used in chinning, climbing a rope, rock and mountain climbing, in raising the body on various pieces of gymnastics apparatus (high bar, parallel bars, unevens), and in various

obstacle course walls. Wrestling and football require this action when grabbing or pulling in an opponent from an outreached position, and it is needed in the martial arts when trying to pull an opponent into position for a throw. In basketball it is needed when pulling the ball in from a high rebound.

The early range of motion is especially important in athletics, particularly in doing explosive movements. It is in this range that the muscle literally explodes, and then the movement goes through the remaining range on inertia.

For bodybuilders, early range development is needed to produce a longer and fuller muscle. Working in this early range is also needed to maintain maximum flexibility in the elbow joint.

Execution

The biceps curl exercise using a barbell will be described to serve as the basic variant for proper execution of the beginning range of motion.

Assume a well-balanced standing position with your feet approximately shoulder-width

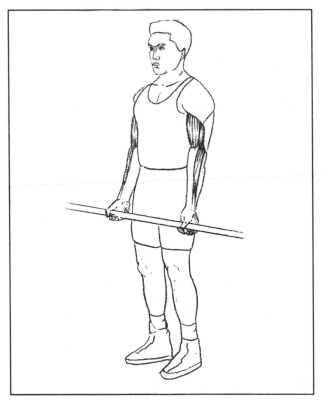

Figure 8.4
Muscles used in the standing biceps curl

apart. Hold a barbell (or an E-Z Curl Bar) in your hands with a supinated (palms facing upward) grip with your hands slightly less than shoulder-width apart. Extend your arms fully so that your elbows are free of or lightly touching the sides of your body. Keep your chest high and your shoulders back and rest the barbell across your upper thighs (see Photo 8.1).

When you are ready, inhale slightly more than usual and hold your breath as you raise the barbell with strong elbow joint flexion. Keep your shoulders and elbows in position at all times while doing the exercise. Raise the bar until your forearms are parallel to the floor and there is approximately a 90-degree angle in your elbows (see Photo 8.2). After reaching this position, begin to exhale and lower the bar under control to the starting fully extended arm position. Allow your arms to relax slightly for a moment and then repeat.

Comments

- When you use very heavy weights, you will have a strong tendency to lean backward and push your pelvic girdle forward to get the weight moving. You should not lean backward in this variant (this is cheating!) because doing so will overcome resting inertia, as a result of which the bar will be put into motion without the strong use of the muscles involved. More importantly, leaning backward creates a tendency to bring your elbows up, which decreases the effective resistance greatly (the weight is not lifted directly against gravity). Leaning backward is usually done for mid-range development of the biceps and brachialis, but because there are many other exercises that work the mid-range more effectively, you should not cheat in this exercise.
- When your arm is straight, the angle of pull of the biceps is very weak. Almost all the force of the flexor muscles pulls the forearm into the upper arm, and only a small amount of residual force is used for rotating the forearm. However, as the forearm moves closer to the horizontal position, the angle of pull changes dramatically. When the angle of pull is 90 degrees (when your forearm is close to the parallel position), the entire biceps muscle is being used to lift the forearm and the weights and there are no stabilization forces (forces that pull into the elbow). Because of this you are much stronger when your arm approaches

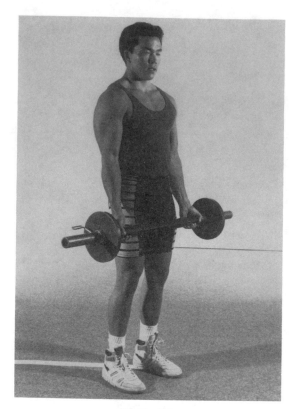

Photo 8.1

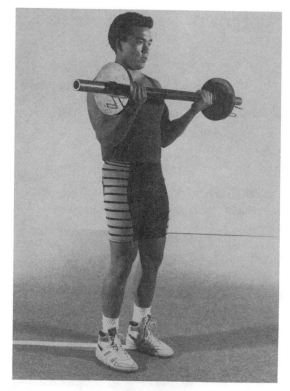

Photo 8.2

the 90-degree angle, and the weight that seemed heavy when your arms were straight appears quite light. Thus, for maximum development of the muscle through the full range of motion, you should work it in sections.

- If you have difficulty keeping your trunk erect with your shoulders, back, and elbows alongside your body, do the exercise standing with your buttocks and shoulders against a wall. This will help prevent you from throwing your hips forward or your shoulders back. In addition, try to touch the wall with your elbows as you perform the exercise. This will teach you to keep your elbows back as needed for proper execution.

- The brachioradialis muscle, in addition to being involved in elbow joint flexion, also acts as a supinator when the hand is pronated and as a pronator when the hand is supinated. Therefore, to elicit a maximal contraction of the brachioradialis, you must use a neutral grip. To do this, you must execute the exercise using dumbbells.

- For many individuals the most effective grip for strong involvement of the biceps brachii is the neutral grip. In this position the biceps has a straight line of pull, and the tendency to supinate from this position is not great. To use a neutral grip, substitute dumbbells for the barbell. Or, you can use the E-Z Curl Bar, which allows you to assume a grip between the neutral and supinated positions. This is very effective for muscle development.

- The brachialis muscle is a true elbow joint flexor. Because it attaches to the ulna, it is equally effective regardless of whether your hand is pronated, supinated, or in a neutral position and is therefore sometimes considered the "workhorse" of the elbow joint flexors. In addition, it is almost as strong as the biceps brachii and plays an important role in the early range of movement.

■ Mid-Range Biceps Curl with a Roto-Bar

The biceps curl with a Roto-Bar (which allows hand rotation against resistance) is one of the best exercises for the biceps muscle in mid-range (the Roto-Bar is shown in Photos 8.3 and 8.4). The reason for this is that it is the only exercise that works the biceps in its two actions: elbow joint flexion and supination. All other biceps exercises involve only one of these actions.

When you execute a biceps curl using very heavy weights, it is impossible to initiate the exercise with your arms held straight. However, heavy weights are sometimes necessary to produce maximum intensity for strength and mass. Because of this, you should begin the exercise with your elbows slightly flexed as in Roto-Bar curls, preacher curls, concentration curls, low pulley curls, and most biceps curl machines. These are very effective exercises, but do not do them to the exclusion of other exercises or you will produce excessive shortening of the muscles.

The Roto-Bar or Keiser biceps curl machine can also be used solely with a supinated or neutral grip. Both of these grips are very effective for development of the elbow joint flexors, and the biceps in particular.

Major muscles and actions involved

The same as for the beginning range bicep curl except the mid-range version allows for a greater range of muscle action (see Figure 8.5).

Sports uses

The same as for the beginning range biceps curl.

Execution

Stand up and assume a well-balanced position with your feet approximately shoulder-width apart. Hold a Roto-Bar in your hands, using a neutral grip to grasp the handles (so that the hand grips are vertical). To maintain this position you may have to flex your wrists radially—raise the thumb side of your hand somewhat so that the grips are vertical. Your arms (forearms) should be flexed approximately 20 degrees at the elbow joint with your elbows alongside your trunk (see Photo 8.3).

When you are ready, inhale and hold your breath as you curl the bar upward. As you approach the 90-degree angle at your elbow joint, supinate your hands (turn your palms upward) and continue the upward motion. There should be no stopping in the lifting movement. Continue the movement until your forearms are above the parallel position (see Photo 8.4). After reaching the upper position where the resistance decreases, exhale and relax your muscles slight-

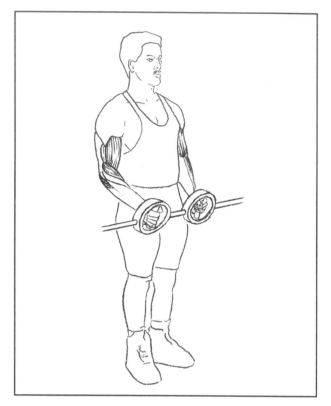

Figure 8.5
Mucles used in the biceps curl with a Roto-Bar

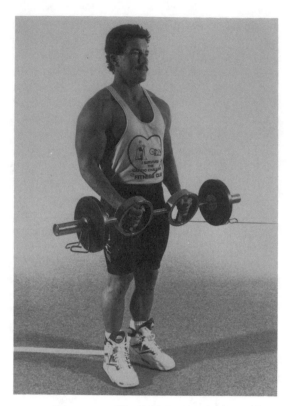

Photo 8.3

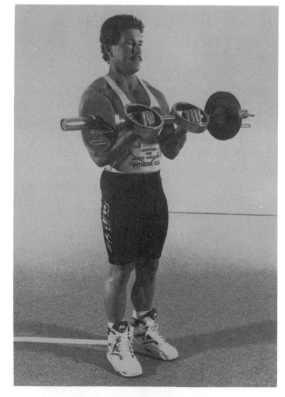

Photo 8.4

ly as you return to the initial position under control. Pronate (turn your palms inward) as you return to the initial position. When you are at the bottom position, quickly inhale and reverse directions to execute the repetitions.

Comments

- This exercise is most effective for the mid-range action of the biceps, where the muscle is most powerful. The Roto-Bar allows you to turn your hands in a supinating action against resistance as you do the exercise. The greater the weight you use, the greater is the resistance as you turn your hands. So, in this exercise the biceps is taxed doubly, not only in the flexion movement, but also in its very important action of supination. This is why using the Roto-Bar is so effective.
- Many bodybuilders try to include shoulder flexion with elbow flexion to create a stronger contraction. This can be done, but only after the biceps is maximally shortened. Thus, do the exercise as described, but upon reaching

the uppermost position, raise your elbow until your arm is horizontal.

- The biceps brachii is a two-joint muscle (shoulder and elbow) because of its attachment to the scapula and the radius. Therefore, in order to get total development of this muscle, it should be worked in both the shoulder and elbow joints. Contraction of the short head is involved in shoulder joint flexion, abduction, inward rotation, and horizontal adduction. Contraction of the long head pulls the humerus into the glenoid cavity, stabilizes movement in the joint, and may assist with abduction.

- For variety you can use the Double-Roto (which is similar to the Roto-Bar but the grips are closer together) on a low pulley system. Place your hands slightly narrower than shoulder-width apart and execute the same way as when using the Roto-Bar.

- In this exercise it is important to keep your upper body erect with your shoulders back. Leaning forward actually gives more slack to the biceps tendons that insert in the shoulder. Most effective is to keep these tendons taut, and to do this you must keep your elbows alongside or behind your body at all times. For maximum stretch of the upper end of the biceps, you can also do lying or incline dumbbell curls. To execute, lie face up on an exercise bench or sit on an incline bench with your arms lowered behind your back. Execute the dumbbell biceps curl while keeping your elbows in the rear position throughout the exercise.

- Because this exercise is mainly for the mid-range of the biceps, you should not strive to extend your arms completely at the bottom position or to flex your arms completely at the top position. By flexing your arms at the top, because of the greater weight, not only will you have to bring your elbows forward, but you will have to turn the Roto attachment in a manner that causes it to lose its effectiveness.

- Breathing plays a very important role in this exercise. First, it allows you to gain greater force when doing the movement so you can use more weights. Second, holding your breath creates greater thoracic and intra-abdominal pressure, which helps hold your spine in place and allows you to maintain a more upright position. This, in turn, allows you to isolate the muscular action to the arm flexors. Third, the correct breathing pattern allows the muscles

to contract and relax to prevent excessive residual muscle tension.

- You should not use your upper body or your legs to start the movement. With the correct weight, there will be immediate muscle tension when you begin the movement. Keep in mind that you are not starting in the bottom position, and therefore the angle of muscle pull of the biceps is more favorable, which allows you to handle more weight in this area without any additional changes in execution. Also keep in mind that the more you use your body to help get the movement started, the less is the effect on the muscles you want to develop.

- The brachioradialis muscle, in addition to being involved in elbow joint flexion, also acts as a supinator when the hand is in a pronated position and as a pronator when the hand is in a supinated position. Therefore, to elicit a maximal contraction of this muscle, a neutral (or pronated) grip must be used. (Note that with the pronated grip you will be doing the reverse biceps curl at the start of the exercise.) Thus, the brachioradialis is strongly involved in two actions in the early part of the movement. However, when the hands are supinated, the brachioradialis is only moderately involved and you must rely on the biceps and brachialis muscles.

- For maximum isolation of the biceps in mid-range, you should do preacher curls, in which you place your upper arm on an incline bench to eliminate any action in the shoulder joints. However, it is important that you do not fully extend your arms when you have great weights because the weights can hyperextend the elbow and cause problems. You should, therefore, keep your elbow bent in the bottom position. One of the better exercises that involves this execution is the biceps curl done on the Keiser biceps machine.

■ Mid-Range Biceps Curl on a Machine

Biceps curl exercise machines can be used to produce effective development of the elbow flexors.

Major muscles and actions involved

The elbow flexors are strongly involved in the mid-range of this exercise and to some extent in the ending range (see Figure 8.6). In this exercise the forearm moves toward the upper arm, which is fully stabilized.

Sports uses

The same as for the beginning range biceps curl.

Execution

The execution will be described on a Keiser machine, but it is basically the same as other biceps exercise machines. Adjust the seat on the machine so that when you are sitting down your shoulders are above the incline pad for placement of the upper arm (similar to the preacher curl). In the final position you should be able to sit upright with your upper arm resting firmly on the pad without any discomfort. If you find yourself leaning in too far, adjust the chest pad to hold yourself in the upright position.

When you are in position, grasp the handles of the resistance lever arms, keeping your elbows slightly bent (see Photo 8.5). You will note that the handles spin freely so that you can assume either a supinated or a neutral grip; rotate your hands as you do the exercise. Also note that the machine can be used unilaterally or with both arms at the same time. If you desire the unilateral movement, pull out the pin that

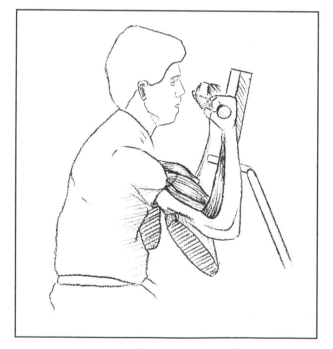

Figure 8.6
Muscles used in the machine biceps curl

locks both bars in place. As you hold the handles of the resistance lever arms, adjust the air pressure to the required amount.

When you are ready, inhale and hold your breath as you bend your elbows and bring your forearms upward. Keep your head directly in the middle of your hands so that the action is in line with your shoulders. After going past the position in which your elbows form a 90-degree angle (see Photo 8.6), exhale as you return under control to the original position. In the bottom position you should maintain a slight angle (10–20 degrees) in the elbow joint to make the beginning of the next repetition easier. Repeat for the desired number of repetitions with both arms together or alternating them, one at a time.

Comments

- The Keiser machine gives maximum isolation of the body and arm when you are properly positioned. Thus, when you do the exercise, all the action takes place at the elbow. However, in this version it is important not to fully extend your arms when they are in the bottom position, especially if your elbows are slightly beyond the edge of the arm pad, because doing so may make you hyperextend your elbow joint, which can strain the muscles and the joint.
- Because the button to change resistance is in the grip, you can easily adjust the amount of resistance throughout the full range of motion. Usually, once the resistance is set, you should not make any changes as you do the repetitions. For variety, however, you can increase the resistance at the beginning range or more in the ending range. However, in the ending range you will have to lift your elbows off the pad, which is usually not recommended except after you have completely flexed your elbows.
- Because of the ease of resistance and adjustability, you can do this exercise at a rapid rate of speed. However, if you do so, the exercise should be done alternating arms so that each arm gets a slight amount of rest between repetitions.
- The ability to supinate your hands in this exercise makes the exercise feel more natural through its full range of motion. However, your hands are not turned against resistance as they are in the Roto-Bar variant.
- When you are using extremely great resistance, it is advisable to do the exercise with both arms

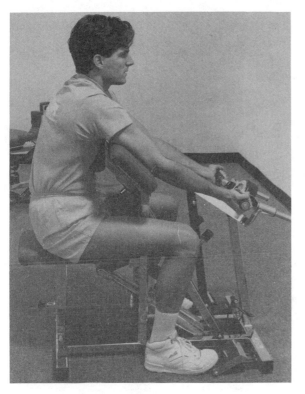

Photo 8.5

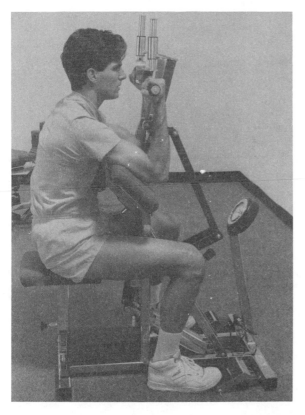

Photo 8.6

simultaneously. In this manner you can maximally stabilize your trunk and create greater force to overcome the resistance. If you do the exercise with only one arm, your body will have a tendency to slide out to one side for more help, and this can be dangerous.

■ Ending Range Biceps Curl with an Iso Bar

With conventional barbells and dumbbells, the biceps can be worked effectively through only a 90-degree range of motion, that is, from when your arm is perfectly straight to when your forearm is perpendicular to your upper arm. When you go beyond this perpendicular position, there is a decrease in effective resistance because the arm movement is no longer done directly against gravity but is made in a more horizontal direction as gravity pulls your arm toward you. Also, when you go beyond 90 degrees, some of the muscle force is used to pull the bones out of the joint rather than move the weight.

To counteract these effects, a specialized bar called the Iso Bar can be used (the Iso Bar is pictured in Photos 8.7 and 8.8). This bar has a double sleeve that allows the arm movement to continue against resistance past the 90-degree angle; the Iso Bar creates additional resistance through the upper range by changing the position of the weights. Because of this the Iso Bar is very effective in peaking, that is, producing maximum shortening of the biceps muscle with maximum height.

Major muscles and actions involved

When doing the biceps curl with the Iso Bar, elbow joint flexion occurs beginning when the elbows are slightly flexed and ending when they are flexed maximally (see Figure 8.7).

Sports uses

The sports uses are essentially the same as those with the exercises that involve the midrange. However, because the Iso Bar is maximally effective in the ending range, this exercise is especially important for wrestlers who often find their arm in this position when holding, for climbers who need a full-range pull, and for arm wrestlers when they are holding their position and trying to push their opponent's forearm

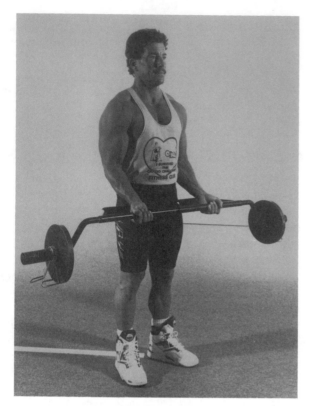

Photo 8.7

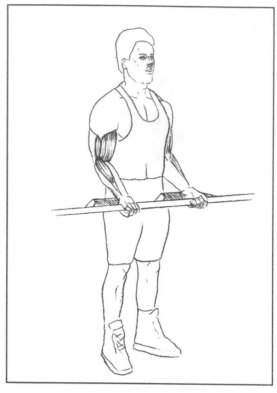

Figure 8.7
Muscles used in the Iso Bar curl

downward. The exercise's greatest value is in the maximum development of the biceps muscle.

Execution

Execution in the early range of motion is exactly the same as with the barbell from a bent-arm position (see Photo 8.7). However, when using the Iso Bar you continue the movement through a maximum range of motion in the ending range (see Photo 8.8). Thus, you should keep pulling (flexing the elbow) until the mass of your biceps contacts your forearm and stops further movement.

Comments

• The Iso Bar begins working when the lift reaches 57 degrees from a vertical start position for the biceps curl. As the bar is lifted, the weights pivot and your forearm braces against the padded lever. As the curl continues upward, the biceps have weight resistance all the way through the lift. Because of this the exercise is maximally effective in the development of muscle mass and especially biceps peaking.

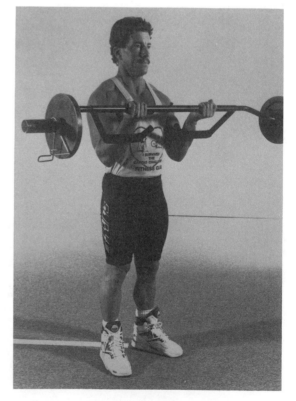

Photo 8.8

- Because the Iso Bar is mostly effective in the middle and ending range, you can use more weight than in the beginning or middle range exercises. However, if you do so, start with your arms bent approximately 45 degrees to the vertical. You will then notice that the exercise is as difficult above as it is below the 90-degree elbow joint angle.

ELBOW JOINT EXERCISES: TRICEPS EXERCISE VARIANTS

Triceps exercises function in a similar manner to the biceps exercises. Some of them are very effective in the early range of motion, which especially involves the medial and lateral heads, and additionally these exercises involve the long head when the stress is on the ending range of motion as the arm becomes fully extended.

There are many different exercises for the triceps. Not only do they require different pieces of equipment, but also a multitude of different handles for different grips and hand positions. Thus you can use a V-Bar, hexagonal bars, the Double-Roto Bar, and machine exercises. Some of the exercises, such as the French press, work mainly the early range of motion, whereas others work the latter range of motion as, for example, the lying 45-degree triceps extension.

■ Beginning Range of Motion French Press

Major muscles and actions involved

In the French (triceps) press the triceps brachii muscle is involved in elbow joint extension (see Figure 8.8). In this action the forearm moves away from the upper arm to a fairly straight arm position.

Sports uses

Elbow joint extension and the muscles involved are very important in execution of many sports skills. For example, they are needed in many overhead hitting actions such as the tennis serve and smash and basketball shooting. Elbow joint extension is a key action in pushing as used in the shot put, pressing up into a handstand in gymnastics, and in hand-to-hand balancing, pushing an opponent in football, and so on.

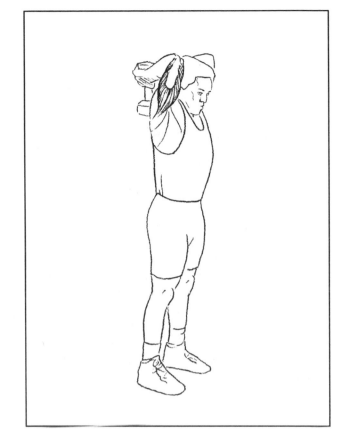

Figure 8.8
Muscles used in the French press

In bodybuilding, development of the triceps in the beginning range of motion is needed for development of the underside of the upper arm, especially the lower and middle portions.

Execution

Stand up with your feet shoulder-width apart and with your body erect and held firm. Hold a dumbbell on one end with both hands with your arms fully extended overhead. Your fingers should be interlaced under the end of the dumbbell (see Photo 8.9).

When you are ready, inhale and hold your breath as you lower the dumbbell under control behind your head as far as possible. Keep your elbows pointed upward (vertical) as you bend your elbows to lower your hands.

When you reach the bottom position (see Photo 8.10), immediately raise the weight back to the starting (overhead) position via elbow joint extension. Keep your elbows pointed straight up throughout the entire up movement. Exhale as you pass the most difficult portion of the lift. Pause momentarily and then repeat.

Comments

- The French press can also be done holding a dumbbell in each hand and executing as you would with one dumbbell, or you can alternate hands. If you alternate hands, you can also pronate your hand at the end of the action. In so doing you can raise your arm higher and place a slightly different stress on the triceps. To extend your arm even higher, you should bend your spine sideways and include greater shoulder elevation. This variant is important for sports that require maximum reaching and for developing greater coordination and other muscles. Also, using the arms singly places less stress on the spine.

- It is very important to keep your elbow pointed straight up. If it drops down in front, it will weaken the action of the triceps tremendously because the weight will no longer produce effective resistance, that is, be lifted directly against gravity.

- For maximal development, you do not have to extend your arms fully. When your arms are bent at a 90-degree angle, the triceps is strongest. Thus, after you pass the 90-degree range, the triceps is no longer very strongly involved. Also, if you fully extend your arms, especially when using heavy weights, there will be compression forces on the elbow joint which could cause injury. In addition, it is important to understand that the medial head of the triceps does most of the work, especially at the beginning of the movement. Therefore, full extension is not needed for development of this portion of the muscle.

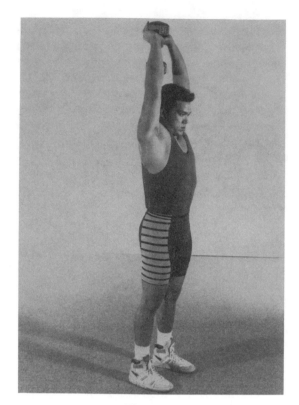

Photo 8.9

■ Mid-Range Triceps Push-Down

One of the best exercises for development of the triceps in mid-range is the triceps push-down with the Double-Roto grip. Other attachments such as the straight bar or V-shaped bar can also be used, but they do not allow for rotation of the hands.

Major muscles and actions involved

The same as in the French press (see Figure 8.9).

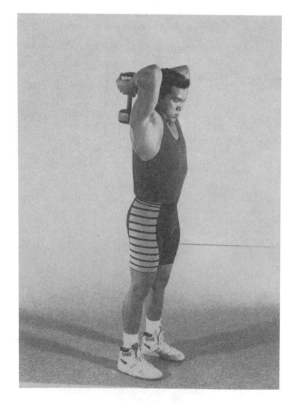

Photo 8.10

Sports uses

The same as for the French press. In addition, mid-range elbow joint extension plays a major role in baseball batting (just prior to ball contact) and in the racquetball, tennis, and badminton backhand strokes. It is extremely important in the martial arts (karate, wrestling, and so on) and for boxers in punching. This is the action that produces up to one-third of the total force in a punch. Also, elbow extension is the key action for arm quickness in reaching.

The triceps push-down is critical in the iron sports, for example, in the jerk in weightlifting and in the bench press in powerlifting. This exercise is also very important for bodybuilders for developing the entire back of the upper arms.

Execution

Stand up in a well-balanced position with your feet slightly wider than shoulder-width apart, or with a slight stride. Position yourself in front of a high pulley with a Double-Roto attachment and

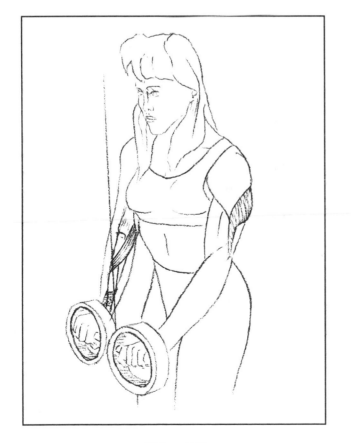

Figure 8.9
Muscles used in the mid-range triceps push-down

grasp the Roto handles with a neutral grip, placing your elbows alongside your body. There should be slightly less than 90 degrees of flexion in the elbow joint (see Photo 8.11).

When you are ready, inhale and hold your breath as you push down with your hands and extend your elbows. Hold your elbows in place, keep your grip firm, and keep your hand and forearm in a straight line as you pull down. Continue extending your elbows, and as you approach the bottom position, turn (pronate) your hands inward until your arms are approximately 10–20 degrees shy of full extension (see Photo 8.12). After reaching this position, relax your muscles somewhat, return to the original position, and repeat.

Comments

- By keeping your wrist and forearm in line with each other, you do not allow your wrist to drop back (hyperextend) as it does when you use the regular straight bar, ropes, or V-shaped attachments. Therefore, you keep the assistant elbow joint extensors (which are wrist extensors) more on stretch so that they can better stabilize the elbow joint and play a role in elbow extension. Because of this, you will find it possible to use more weight to create more tension, with the resulting greater development of muscle strength and/or mass.
- By incorporating hand pronation near the end of elbow extension, you will experience a much stronger contraction than when you use other cable attachments. When you pronate your hand (under resistance), you slightly displace the ulna bone, to which the triceps attaches, thereby producing a different angle of pull. This is why you will find the upper head of the triceps kicking in very strongly along with the middle and lateral heads. As an added benefit, you develop the assistant elbow extensors and pronator muscles of the forearm. Also, keep in mind that the wrist extensors (and flexors) remain under a strong isometric contraction to hold the wrist in place.
- The key to pure isolation of muscle action is to maintain your elbows in a position close to the sides of your body or in front of your body. You can stand back a little in order to place your elbows in front of you, but it is essential that they do not move. If you use shoulder joint extension and pull your elbows back as you begin the elbow joint extension, you will be

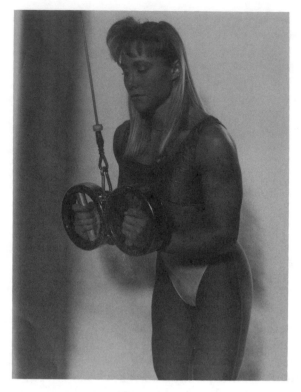

Photo 8.11

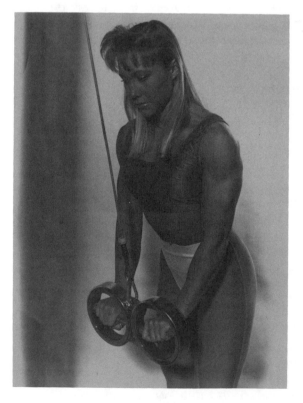

Photo 8.12

cheating. In this variant you will be using your shoulder joint extensors to get the movement started and bringing in elbow joint extension when the inertia (resistance) is not as great.

Keeping your elbows out in front puts the long head of the triceps on stretch, which creates a stronger contraction. This is especially noticeable near the end of the movement, but only if you keep your elbows in position. When you stand slightly away from the grip, as when you use a stride position, it is important that you do not use your upper trunk to get the weight started moving. Your upper body must remain in place and not drop down, especially as you begin the exercise. If your upper body drops, you will be using the momentum of your body to assist in the exercise, which takes stress off the triceps.

- It should also be noted that the narrow grip made possible by the Double-Roto or other attachments contributes to greater effectiveness in working the triceps. When the grip is narrow, it places greater stress on the triceps in addition to allowing you to go through a greater range of motion. The Double-Roto is the most advanced technological development for maximum triceps involvement. However, other grips are available which can be used for variety. For example, you can use a hexagonal shaped bar, which has a two-inch diameter that allows you to keep your fingers more open and your hand more in line with your forearm. Also available is a one- and two-inch diameter V-bar with a wide flange at the base so that the heel of your hand can rest against it. This allows you to relax your grip, which enables you to concentrate harder on using the triceps.
- An effective variant for development of the triceps in the mid-range is the overhead triceps cable press. In this exercise you bend over from the hips so that your trunk is fairly parallel to the floor, and then you pull a high cable from behind your head to in front of your head via elbow extension. Your arms should not be fully extended, however, because of potentially high compression forces on the elbow.

■ Mid-Range Triceps Extension on a Machine

Most triceps exercises are done at a slow to moderate rate of speed. However, working the muscles at a fast speed is often effective for strength and speed work in mid-range. To do this, use a triceps extension machine such as the one by Keiser.

Muscles and actions involved

In this exercise the triceps is involved in elbow extension as the forearm moves away from the upper arm. There is also some flexion in the shoulder joint, which involves the upper pectoralis major, the anterior deltoid, and the coracobrachialis (see Figure 8.10). In this action the elbow moves from a position behind the body to alongside the body.

Sports uses

The same as for the other triceps exercises and the dip exercise.

Execution

Adjust the seat height so that when you are seated and you grasp the handles of the resistance lever arms, there is a 90-degree or narrower angle in your elbow joint. Grasp the handles with a neutral grip and keep your body in an erect seated position with your eyes looking straight ahead of you (see Photo 8.13). Adjust the resistance by pressing down with your heel.

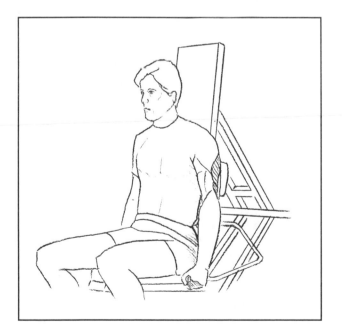

Figure 8.10
Muscles used in the mid-range triceps
extension on a machine

When you are ready, inhale and hold your breath as you begin to push down. Keep pushing until your arms are fully extended (see Photo 8.14). When you reach the bottommost position, exhale slightly and return to the initial position and repeat. Concentrate on elbow extension.

Comments

- Because the triceps extension on the Keiser machine is most effective in the middle and ending range, you should not start in a position with your elbow high and with a very small angle in the elbow joint. Not only does this place extreme pressure on the joints but, even more importantly, it is not the best angle for mid-range development of the triceps.
- The Keiser machine also enables you to do the exercise for speed and quickness. To do this, decrease the usual resistance used for strength and then push your arms down quickly. Do not try for complete elbow extension, however. The fast contraction should occur early in the range of motion, and then the eccentric resistance should slow you down so that you can quickly return to the upward position for another quick reversal of direction.
- When you do quick or explosive actions, the muscular contraction occurs early in the range of motion and then inertia (momentum) carries the limb to full length. Because of this, in a typical weight stack machine, there is no danger of injury as you approach the end position. However, because the Keiser machine uses air, there is *no* momentum and thus no danger of injury when you are doing speed movements. In addition, you can do the triceps extension either unilaterally or alternating your arms to simulate the repetitive actions of the arms in various sports.
- When you use the Keiser machine, you should also use three different muscle contraction regimes for maximum strength. By increasing the resistance at different points of the range of motion on the pushing phase, you can get a greater concentric contraction and then on the return increase the resistance to get a greater eccentric contraction. Also, stop and hold different positions in the range of motion with increased resistance for an isometric (static) contraction. When you do a combination of these three muscle contraction regimes, you can gain even greater strength than when you limit yourself to only one movement, especially

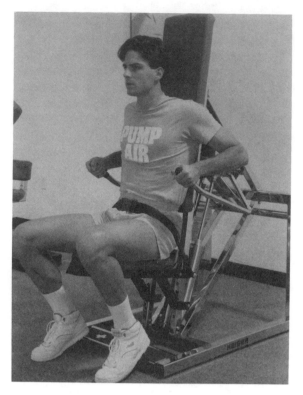

Photo 8.13

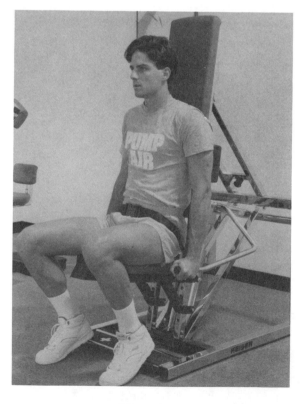

Photo 8.14

the concentric. In addition, you can work at exactly the angles needed in your sport.

- When using the Keiser machine, the triceps muscle is not completely isolated. When you press down there is also shoulder joint flexion similar to what occurs in the dip exercise. For greater depth of movement, you can move your hands back somewhat on the grips so your hands are directly below your shoulders. In this version the spine is kept erect. You can also lower the seat to raise your elbows higher.

- In addition, as far as I know, the Keiser triceps machine is the only machine upon which you can also isolate shoulder girdle depression. To do this, keep your arms straight and firmly in place and then push down with your shoulders. The eccentric return will bring your shoulders back up, and then you must push down and depress them. All these actions take place while you remain in the seated position.

■ End-Range 45-Degree Triceps Extension

To work the ending range of motion in triceps extension, an especially effective exercise for the long head of the triceps and for maximum definition of the entire muscle is the 45-degree triceps extension.

Major muscles and actions involved

The same as in the other triceps exercises (see Figure 8.11). In addition, full extension of the arms makes some activities even more effective.

Sports uses

The same as for the other triceps exercises.

Execution

Lie down in a stable supine position on an exercise bench. Hold a Roto-Bar or dumbbells in your hands with your arms extended and held at a 45-degree angle to the horizontal behind your head. Use a neutral grip, especially when using the Roto-Bar. This is the true ending position. When you are ready, inhale and hold your breath as you bend your elbows and lower your forearms until they hang perpendicular (straight down) behind your head (see Photo 8.15). During the lowering action, be sure to hold your elbows in place. Upon reaching the bottom position,

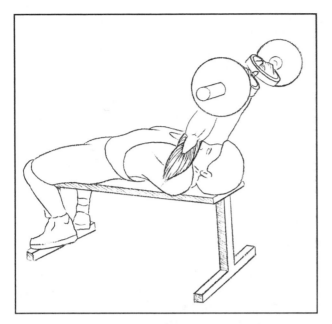

Figure 8.11
Muscles used in the 45-degree triceps extension

lift of the dumbbells. In essence, you will then be doing a pullover, which overcomes the initial inertia of the weights and takes the stress off the triceps. For maximum muscle development, it is important to have full extension of the elbow at the end of the movement. This ending movement is necessary to maximally shorten and tense the lateral and long heads of the triceps. It should also be noted that in this version the compression forces on the elbow are not great.

• The 45-degree triceps extension is very similar to the lying triceps extension, but they are not the same. In the typical lying triceps extension, you must be careful not to hit your head. Also, the lying triceps extension involves more of the beginning or middle ranges of motion.

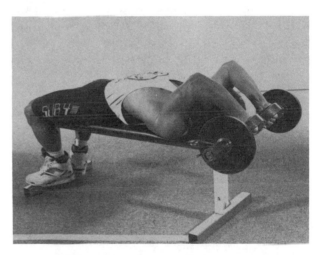

Photo 8.15

vigorously extend your arms in the elbow joints until your elbows are fully extended and held at a 45-degree angle to the horizontal (see Photo 8.16). When using a Roto-Bar, simultaneously pronate your forearms (turn your hands in so your palms face upward). Your upper arm should be held at a 45-degree angle to your body (to the horizontal) at all times. Exhale as you return to the final position and then repeat.

Comments

• It is extremely important that you hold your elbow in position at a 45-degree angle to the horizontal. If you allow it to drop down to the rear, it will change the stress placed on the triceps during the pull. By holding your elbows in position, you place the triceps under greater tension, which, in turn, produces a more powerful contraction. In addition, the long head of the triceps remains under a strong isometric contraction while the Roto-Bar or dumbbells are lowered, which, in turn, produces a stronger concentric contraction during the lift. As a result, you gain greater strength.

• If you drop your elbows, you will have a greater tendency to change the way the exercise is executed. For example, when you drop your elbows, you will raise them again during the

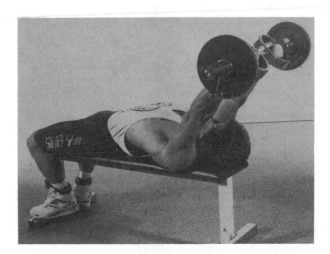

Photo 8.16

■ End-Range Triceps Kickback

Another effective exercise to work the long head in two actions is the triceps kickback (see Figure 8.12).

Execution

Assume a bent-over position so that your trunk is horizontal (parallel to the floor). Your feet should be flat on the floor in a stride or square stance and your knees should be slightly bent. Hold a dumbbell with a neutral grip and bend your arm so that your upper arm is alongside your body and your forearm hangs straight down or is slightly under your arm. Support your body with your free arm by placing your hand on a bench (see Photo 8.17).

When you are ready, inhale slightly more than usual and hold your breath as you extend your arm until it is straight. Keep your elbow in place as you move the hand with the weight backward and upward in an arc of a circle (see Photo 8.18). After your arm is fully extended, continue the upward movement as far as possible. In the final position the dumbbell should be above the level of your back, which should remain parallel to the floor (see Photo 8.19). Exhale and slowly return to the initial position, keeping the weight under control.

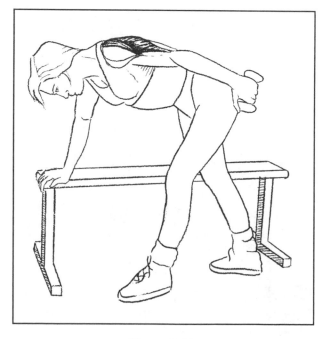

Figure 8.12
Muscles used in the end-range triceps kickback

Comments

- In correct execution you must maintain a stable bent-over position so that your back remains in the horizontal position. This is needed for safety and to ensure that the muscles work directly against gravity for maximum resistance.

- In their zeal to use heavier weights, many athletes and bodybuilders raise their shoulder to get the weight sufficiently up and back. This action uses the spinal rotational muscles and does not fully involve the long head of the triceps. The key is to keep your shoulders in place.

- Excessively heavy weights lead to a decreased range of motion and also limit your ability to fully extend your arm. This defeats the purpose of the exercise and when continued for a long time can decrease your flexibility.

- In comparison to other triceps extension exercises, the triceps kickback is more difficult to execute. It requires more stability, coordination, and balance for effective execution. Therefore, before beginning this exercise you should be proficient in doing other triceps exercises.

- When executing the arm raise portion of this exercise, only the long head of the triceps is actively involved. At the same time, the medial and lateral heads as well as the lower end of the long head remain under isometric contraction to keep the elbow joint extended. As a result, you get a "double" contraction of the long head of the triceps, i.e., at both ends of the muscle. First the lower end shortens and remains contracted while the upper end contracts, providing you with maximal shortening of the muscle. This produces the greatest muscle contraction, which is the key to strength development.

- Many bodybuilders and athletes have a tendency to swing the weight so that they can raise it as high as possible. However, this defeats the purpose of the exercise. When you allow the weight to descend quickly from close to your chest and then continue on back and upward, inertia carries the weight up to the maximum and your muscles do very little work except to guide the action. Because of this, it is important that you stop after your arm is straight and then raise your arm. You will feel a distinct difference when execution is done in this manner.

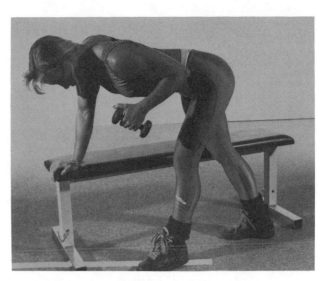

Photo 8.17

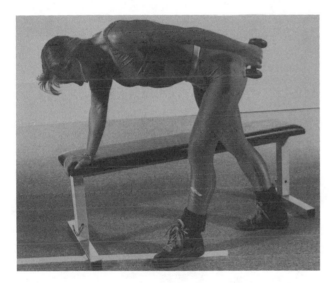

Photo 8.18

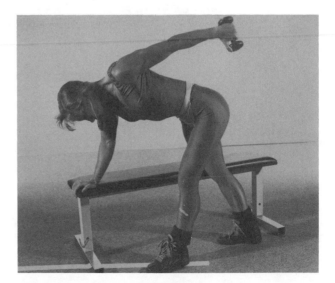

Photo 8.19

9 The Radio-Ulnar Joint

ANATOMY OF THE RADIO-ULNAR JOINT

The radio-ulnar joint is a combination of three joints: the proximal (elbow), middle, and distal (wrist) radio-ulnar joints. The proximal radio-ulnar joint is a pivot joint between the head of the radius and the radial notch of the ulna. The middle radio-ulnar joint is a slightly movable ligamentous joint. The forearm bones are connected by a ligamentous sheath, the interosseous membrane. This membrane prevents undue separation of the two bones, and it acts to transmit and cushion the longitudinal forces of weight bearing. For example, when the arm is in a supporting position, the body weight is transferred from the humerus primarily to the ulna, and the force of resistance from the hand is transferred primarily to the radius at the wrist joint. The distal radio-ulnar joint is a pivot joint between the distal head of the ulna and the ulna notch of the radius. In pronation and supination, the end of the radius glides around the head of the ulna and rotates on its long axis.

BASIC MOVEMENTS IN THE RADIO-ULNAR JOINT

Only two actions are possible in the radio-ulnar joint: supination and pronation. In supination the forearm is rotated so that the hand is turned palm up. In pronation the forearm is rotated so that the hand is turned palm down.

MAJOR MUSCLES INVOLVED

The pronator teres and the pronator quadratus are involved in pronation. The pronator teres is a small muscle that lies across the elbow in front and is partially covered by the brachioradialis. It has two heads, one attached to the epicondyle of the humerus and the other to the coronoid process of the ulna. At the other end the muscle inserts on the lateral surface of the radius near its center. The pronator quadratus is composed of a square sheet of parallel fibers lying deep on the front of the forearm near the wrist. It originates on the lower fourth of the anterior surface of the ulna and inserts on the lower fourth of the anterior surface of the radius (see Figure 9.1).

In supination, the supinator muscle acts alone in slow or fast movements. The biceps brachii comes into play when supination occurs against resistance or when supination is done quickly with the elbow flexed. The supinator muscle is situated under the brachioradialis (see Figure 9.1). The supinator originates on the lateral epicondyle of the humerus, the supinator crest of the ulna, and the ligaments in between. Insertion is on the outer surface of the upper third of the radius. See Chapter 8 for a description of the biceps.

RADIO-ULNAR JOINT EXERCISES

The exercises effectively develop the supinator and pronator muscles are supination and prona-

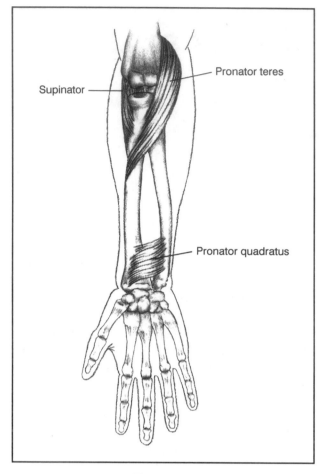

Figure 9.1
Anterior view of the lower right arm

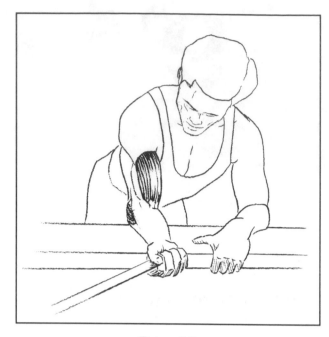

Figure 9.2
Muscles used in supination

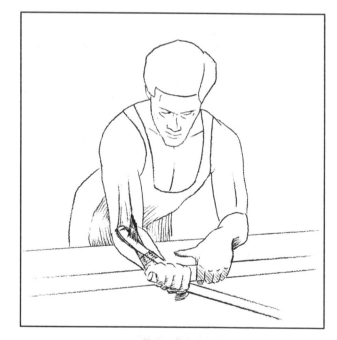

Figure 9.3
Muscles used in pronation

tion with the Strength Bar, supination and pronation with the Roto-Bar, and supination and pronation with the wrist roller. These will be described briefly.

■ Supination–Pronation with the Strength Bar

Major muscles and actions involved

The supinator and biceps are involved in supination, whereas the pronator quadratus and the pronator teres are involved in pronation (see Figures 9.2 and 9.3).

In supination the palm of the hand is turned upward while the elbow is kept bent at a 90-degree angle, and in pronation the palm of the hand is turned downward while the elbow is kept bent at a 90-degree angle.

Sports uses

Of the two movements, pronation is more important in most sports actions. However, to keep the muscles in balance, the supinators must also be adequately developed. Pronation is used in almost all hitting and throwing actions, for example, in baseball pitching, football throwing, baseball and softball batting, racquet sports forehands and overheads, and in the golf hit.

Supination plays an important role in backhand strokes in the racquet sports, in baseball and softball batting, and in other backhand actions. Supination is also very important in throwing curves in underhand softball pitching. It is also most important for bodybuilders in developing the forearm mass and the biceps brachii. Pronation develops only the forearm and provides for more effective triceps development.

Bodybuilding and weight training exercises do not include supination or pronation when a barbell is used. The reason for this is that with a barbell, the hands are in a locked position. However, in many exercises you should supinate or pronate to allow your hands to move more naturally and safely.

Execution

Supination and pronation can be done separately or at the same time. For convenience, they will be described as one exercise.

Kneel in front of the long side of an exercise bench. Place one of your forearms across the bench seat so that your wrist and hand are clear of the seat. Hold a Strength Bar (12–15 inches long) in your hand in a neutral grip—that is, with your thumb uppermost, the bar vertical, and the weight at the top end. This is the starting position (see Photo 9.1).

When you are ready, turn your hand palm down until the shaft of the bar is level with the bench or slightly below it if you have good flexibility (see Photo 9.2). Keep your forearm and elbow in contact with the bench, and then turn your hand palm up and over so that once again the shaft of the Strength Bar is level with the bench or slightly below it (see Photo 9.3). Repeat, alternating left and right sides for the necessary number of repetitions. Keep your shoulder over your elbow so that you maintain a 90-degree angle in the elbow at all times and so that the elbow remains in contact with the bench. Repeat with the other hand.

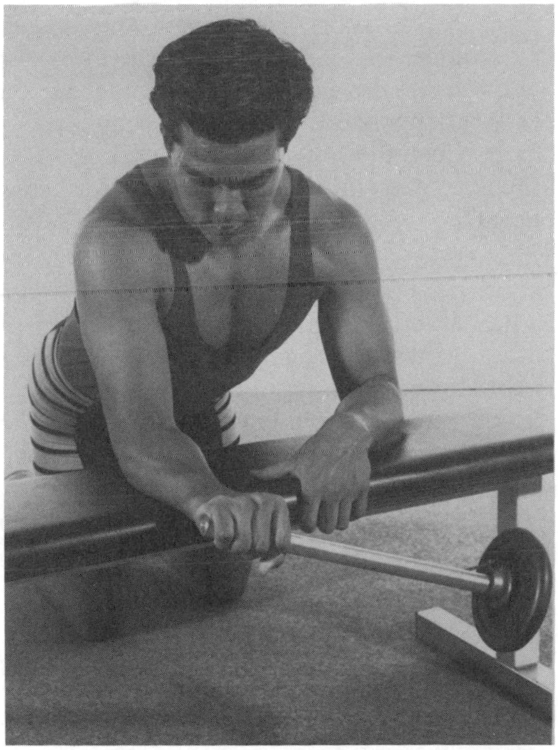

Comments

- Supination–pronation can also be done with a dumbbell. However, it is not very effective

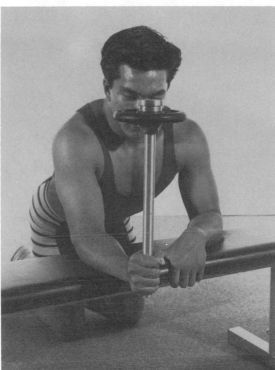

Photo 9.1

Photo 9.2

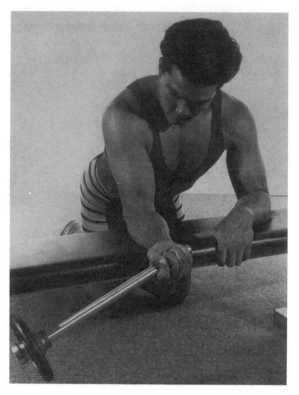

Photo 9.3

shoulders, or out in front. You then rotate the Strength Bar or Roto-Bar handles clockwise and counterclockwise, holding your arms stationary to develop the muscles in both joints. These are very good exercises for pitchers and tennis players, who sometimes injure the rotator muscles.

• The Strength Bar is very similar to the Thor's hammer. However, the Thor's hammer is limited in use. The Strength Bar has a sleeve for both two-inch and one-inch plates and has greater leverage so you do not have to use as much weight on the end. Because of its length, the Strength Bar is very suitable for use by tennis and golf players to develop the forearm muscles as needed in their respective sports. In addition, supination and pronation exercises are very important in preventing various athletic injuries such as pitcher's arm, tennis elbow, and golfer's elbow.

• The key to success in this exercise is the range of motion with your forearm held stationary. Thus, your forearm must remain in place at all times and your elbows must not rise up. Also, your forearm should rotate sufficiently to allow the bar to come to a position that is parallel to the floor. For some athletes, especially pitchers, the range of motion should be even greater.

• Because relatively small weights (usually 2.5 to 5 pounds) are used in this exercise, especially when using the longest radius of the Strength Bar, breathing does not play a critical role. However, when you become fatigued or if you use very heavy weights, then you should inhale and hold your breath during the raising action in both supination and pronation. Exhale as you approach the vertical position in preparation for either one of these actions. Holding your breath will help to stabilize your body and allow you to create greater force to be able to handle the weights safely and effectively.

when done this way because the resistance lever arm is short. In essence, the closer the resistance, the easier it is to turn your hand and the less development that can occur. However, when you are using the Strength Bar, you can adjust the length of the lever by holding the weighted end closer to or farther from your hand.

• Also effective is the use of a Roto-Bar, which allows for supination and pronation under adjustable resistance in many different positions. However, to isolate the supinators and pronators, you must maintain your elbow at a 90-degree angle and execute supination and pronation with your forearm while you are either standing or seated.

• For an even greater range of motion (up to 280 degrees), supination–pronation can be done with your arms held straight with the Strength Bar or Roto-Bar. When done this way, the medial and lateral rotators in the shoulder joint are also involved, which produces the greater range of motion. For example, you can assume a standing position with your arms straight, parallel to the floor, in line with your

■ Power Roller (Wrist Roller) Exercise

Most exercises require movement in a vertical or horizontal plane, which means that the limbs move in only one direction. However, when you use your hands and arms in sports and other activities, they do a multitude of actions across all planes. Therefore, it is important to duplicate

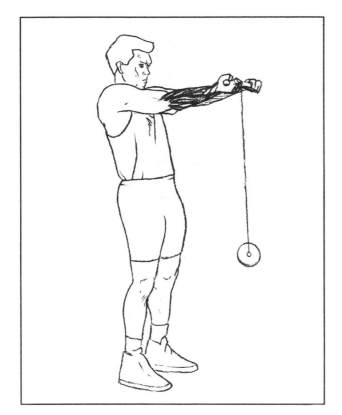

Figure 9.4
Muscles used in the Power Roller exercise

that Variant 3, in which a combination of movements is done, is very effective for the prevention of tennis and golf elbow. In addition, when you use the one-inch Power Roller, you can also do the exercises for speed to develop quick reacting muscles in the forearm. This cannot be done with regular weights because of the probability of injury from the momentum developed.

Execution

Variant 1: In this variant you can do the exercise with a supinated or pronated grip. If you wish to develop your flexors, use a supinated grip; if you wish to develop your extensors, use a pronated grip. Stand up with your arms straight in front of you and parallel to the floor. Grasp the ends of the Power Roller so that the line holding the weight is hanging straight down and taut. The string should be on the inside of the bar (between the bar and your chest). Keep your arms in a straight position and execute wrist flexion and extension in a curling action to roll up the string on the roller pipe (see Photo 9.4). When the weight reaches the uppermost position, unroll the string under muscular control (eccentric contraction).

some of these movements with strength exercises. The best exercises are ones done using the Power Roller (wrist roller).

There are several variants of the wrist roller exercise. In Variant 1 the wrists undergo flexion and extension–hyperextension. In Variant 2 forearm supination and pronation occur. Variant 3 is a combination of 1 and 2. All of these actions are described in the sections on wrist flexion–extension and supination–pronation.

Major muscles and actions involved

The same as in ulna-radial flexion, supination–pronation, and wrist flexion and extension, all of which are discussed in this chapter or in Chapter 10 (also see Figure 9.4).

Sports uses

The sports in which these movements are needed are the same as those described in wrist flexion–extension, supination–pronation, and ulna-radial flexion. However, using a combination of movements is sometimes very beneficial in injury prevention. For example, I have found

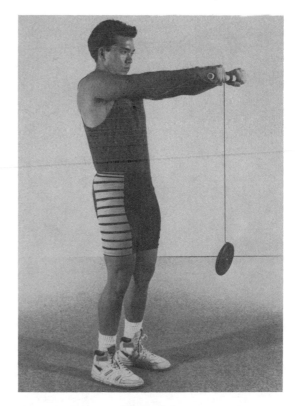

Photo 9.4

Variant 2: In this version you must use a pronated grip. Stand up with your arms parallel to the floor and slightly bent at the elbows, which are pointed out to the sides (see Photo 9.5). Begin with the string taut and execute supination and pronation (turn your hands palm up and palm down) to roll up the string. When the weight reaches the uppermost position, unroll the string using your forearms and hands in the same actions as when rolling up but with the reverse muscle force.

Variant 3: In this variant of the wrist roll, assume a pronated grip with your arms parallel to the floor but with your elbows bent at approximately a 90- to 100-degree angle at the elbow (see Photo 9.6). In this position the Power Roller should be fairly close to your chest, and your forearms should be fairly close to being in line with the Power Roller. In this variant you must use a combination of wrist flexion and extension, supination and pronation, and ulna and radial deviation to roll the string up and down.

Comments

- In Variant 1 it is important to keep your arms straight when doing the exercise. If you bend your elbows, you start using other actions such as supination–pronation and ulna-radial flexion.
- For even greater variety, do the exercise with the string close to you and also with the string on the opposite side. You will notice a switching of the muscular force needed to raise and lower the string.
- Two-inch and one-inch diameter Power Roller bars are available. If you have large hands, the two-inch diameter bar is recommended. The reason for this is that when you use a one-inch bar, you must make a fairly tight fist to maintain a good grip on the roller, which, in turn, does not allow you a full range of motion in the wrist joint. With the two-inch bar, the finger muscle-tendons that cross the wrists are more relaxed, which allows for greater mobility.
- When using the one-inch diameter wrist roller at a fast rate of speed, you can also develop the fast reacting muscles in the fingers and forearms. However, you will also notice that you will be unable to continue at a high rate of speed for any appreciable length of time.

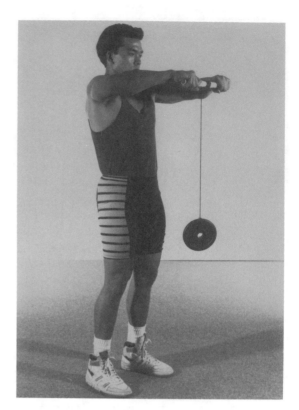

Photo 9.5

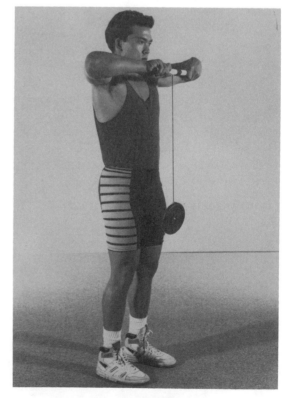

Photo 9.6

10 The Wrist Joint

ANATOMY OF THE WRIST JOINT

There are several "wrist joints." First, there is articulation in the radio-carpal joint formed by the end of the radius bone of the forearm and three of the first row of carpal (wrist) bones (the scaphoid, lunate, and triquetrum). The ulna bone of the forearm does not participate because it is separated from the carpals by a disc of fibrocartilage.

The two rows of carpal bones articulate at the intercarpal joints. The carpal bones glide across one another and allow some flexion and slight extension. Also, the carpal bones in each row articulate with the bone or bones adjacent to them in the same row. Movements of the thumb take place in the carpo-metacarpal joint. Movement of the thumb is atypical because it includes many varied and different movements.

BASIC MOVEMENTS IN THE WRIST JOINT

All movements (except rotation) can occur in the wrist joint. This includes adduction (also known as ulna flexion) in which the little finger side of the hand moves toward the body when the arm is in the anatomical position, that is, when the palm faces forward. The opposite of adduction is abduction, also known as radial flexion, in which the thumb side of the hand moves away from the body when the arm is in the anatomical position.

The wrist can also undergo flexion, in which the palm side of the hand moves toward the forearm. The opposite movement is extension–hyperextension, in which the back of the hand moves toward the posterior surface of the forearm. A combination of all these movements produces circumduction. In this movement, the hand turns around so that the fingers circumscribe a circle and the hand a cone. In many respects the wrist joint is analogous to the ankle joint because it consists of more than one joint with different actions taking place in each joint.

MAJOR MUSCLES INVOLVED

Six principal muscles act on the wrist joint:

1. Flexor carpi radialis—flexion and abduction (radial flexion)
2. Palmaris longus—flexion
3. Flexor carpi ulnaris—flexion and adduction (ulna flexion)
4. Extensor carpi radialis longus—extension and abduction (radial flexion)
5. Extensor carpi radialis brevis—extension and abduction (radial flexion)
6. Extensor carpi ulnaris—extension and adduction (ulna flexion)

Some of the wrist muscles whose masses are located high on the forearm also have finger and elbow joint actions. Close to the wrist the muscles are replaced by long, strong tendons that continue into the hand and provide for less muscle bulk in the wrist and hand, which allows a greater number of muscles to be involved in hand actions.

The flexor carpi radialis and flexor carpi ulnaris contribute much of the muscle mass on the inner front side of the forearm. They have a common tendon for attachment on the inner condyle of the humerus at the upper end. The radialis inserts on the second and third metacarpal bones and the ulnaris on the fifth metacarpal bone (see Figure 10.1). These two muscles are mainly flexors of the wrist and stabilizers of the elbow joint. In addition, the flexor carpi radialis assists in pronation.

The palmaris longus is a slender muscle that lies between the flexor carpi radialis and the flexor carpi ulnaris. It too originates on the inner condyle of the humerus at the upper end, and inserts in the hand. It is a weak elbow flexor and may assist in pronation. This muscle is absent in about 15 percent of the population.

The extensor group of muscles occupies the posterior surface and lateral (outer) border of the forearm. The extensor carpi radialis longus arises just above the lateral condyle of the humerus. The extensor carpi radialis brevis is closely associated with it and arises from the lateral condyle. The two muscles have a common tendon sheath, and the longus inserts on the second metacarpal bone and the brevis on the third metacarpal bone of the hand (see Figure 10.2). Both muscles extend the wrist and forearm.

The extensor carpi ulnaris shares the common extensor tendon at its origin on the lateral condyle of the humerus and inserts on the fifth metacarpal bone of the hand. It is involved in wrist joint extension and stabilization and possibly assists in extension of the elbow.

WRIST JOINT EXERCISES

■ Wrist Curl (Wrist Flexion)

Most bodybuilders, athletes, fitness buffs, and people in general do not perform wrist-strengthening exercises. However, the wrist is involved in a great many activities and is in constant use throughout the day. Because of this, it should be strengthened greatly not only to enhance performance, but also to prevent

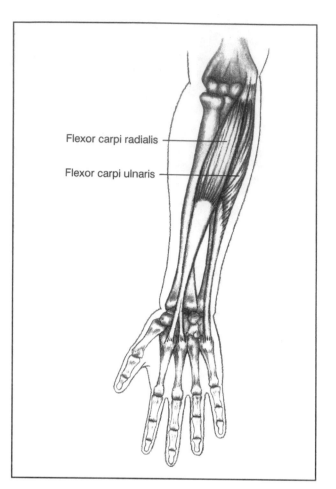

Figure 10.1
Anterior view of the right forearm

injury and to allow you to do other activities more effectively.

For example, stronger wrists enable you to use more weight in other exercises. Doing wrist-strengthening exercises develops the forearms much more than does holding weights in your hands when you perform other exercises. In addition, by strengthening the wrists it is possible to prevent many of the increasingly severe injuries, such as carpal tunnel syndrome, which affect the general population as well as athletes. One of the best exercises to develop the wrist flexors is the wrist curl.

Major muscles and actions involved

The flexor carpi ulnaris and the flexor carpi radialis muscles are involved in wrist joint flexion (see Figure 10.3). In this action the palm side of the hand moves toward the forearm.

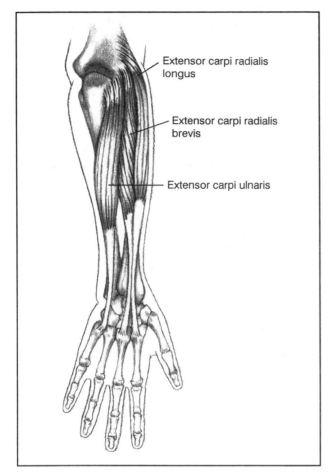

Figure 10.2
Posterior view of the right forearm

in the strength of the muscles involved. Also, wrist flexion is an important action in resisting and dropping the opponent's hand in arm wrestling. For bodybuilders, the wrist curl is a key exercise for developing the inner and outer sides of the forearm.

Execution

The wrist curl is commonly done in a kneeling position with your forearms placed on a bench, or seated with your forearms on your thighs. The kneeling position is preferred because it provides greater stability. Also, the kneeling position allows you to use different equipment, such as the barbell, dumbbell, and Strength Bar. The Strength Bar is preferred when exercising both wrists at the same time because of the centrally located weight and ease of balance.

Kneel in front of an exercise bench placed perpendicular to your body. Place your forearms on the bench with your hands extended beyond the far edge for free movement. Use a supinated grip (palms up) and grasp the ends of the Strength Bar. Keep your shoulders set back somewhat so that your arms are slightly bent.

When you are ready, lower your hands so that your wrist is hyperextended (see Photo 10.1). From this position raise the weight as high as possible (see Photo 10.2). Keep your forearms

Sports uses

Wrist joint flexion and the muscles involved are most important in almost all sports that require throwing actions. These include baseball, football, team handball, softball, javelin, lacrosse, and basketball. In the field events in track, wrist joint flexion is essential in the shot put and javelin throw. It is also very important in hitting actions such as the tennis and racquetball flat serves, smashes, and forehands, and the volleyball spike.

Wrist flexion can also play an important role in many exercises. For example, because the wrist is hyperextended in many overhead lifting exercises, the wrist flexors must be strong to withstand this stress. The wrist (and fingers) must also be sufficiently strong to grip and hold heavy weights without the use of straps, which, if used constantly, eventually lead to a decrease

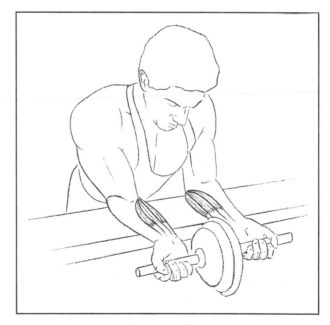

Figure 10.3
Muscles used in the wrist curl with the Strength Bar

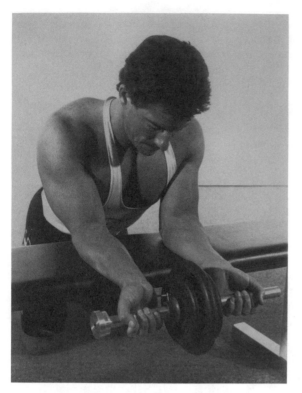

Photo 10.1

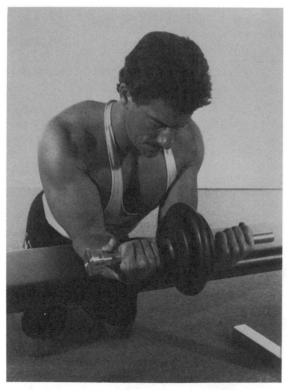

Photo 10.2

on the bench at all times and your body in place. Execute at a moderate rate of speed.

Comments

- To be most effective, the wrist curl should be done through a full range of motion. This means that you should move the weight through approximately 130–160 degrees of motion (65–80 degrees below and 65–80 degrees above the horizontal position). If you are moving the weight far less than this, you are probably using too heavy a weight and therefore not getting full shortening of the muscles. This may lead to a decrease in wrist joint flexibility, which means that you will have weaker execution of various sports skills.
- The flexor carpi radialis and ulnaris muscles cross both the wrist and elbow joints, and they have an action at each end. Therefore, in order to obtain a maximal contraction at the wrist, your elbow must be firmly stabilized. It is also effective to stretch and tense the muscles at the elbow joint by straightening your arms. When the elbow is extended, the tendons of the muscles become taut at the upper end.
- For successful execution, it is very important that you keep your forearm in contact with the bench at all times. Because the flexor muscles also cross the elbow joint, there is a tendency for elbow flexion, which will then bring in other muscles to raise the weight.
- When you use dumbbells, it is important to keep the shaft of the dumbbell in a horizontal position at all times. When the wrist flexors contract, they contract to execute all their actions, and therefore you may find radial or ulna flexion occurring as you do the wrist flexion. You must counteract this, however, by bringing in the opposing muscles to neutralize rotational action and thus get pure wrist flexion. Also, when you use a barbell, some balance is required to hold the barbell level, but with the Strength Bar, there is little need for balance.

■ **Reverse Wrist Curl (Wrist Extension)**

Because wrist flexion is so important in sports and bodybuilding, the extensor muscles are usually ignored. However, the extensors play an important role in maintaining the correct muscle balance at the wrist. In addition, you need well-developed wrist extensors to hold your hand in position while you do many activities with your hand and fingers. To develop the wrist extensors–hyperextensors, then, you should do the reverse wrist curl.

Major muscles and actions involved

The extensor carpi radialis longus and brevis and the extensor carpi ulnaris are involved in wrist joint extension–hyperextension (see Figure 10.4). In this action the back of your hand moves toward your forearm from a flexed position.

Sports uses

The action of wrist joint extension and the muscles involved are most important in the racquet sports when you hit backhand shots. In addition, strong wrist extensors are important for precise movements when you execute wrist and finger flexion. It is important to understand that the main finger extensors are also assistant wrist extensors. If these muscles are weak, you will have difficulty holding your hand in position when doing precise movements with a ball or other object such as a baseball bat or golf club.

Also, the wrist extensors are often needed for the preparatory action to load the wrist flexors before they can act powerfully. In bodybuilding the reverse wrist curl is the main exercise used to develop the outer (posterior) side of the forearm.

Execution

Like the wrist curl, the reverse wrist curl is usually executed in one of two positions—kneeling with your forearms placed on an exercise bench or seated with your forearms on your thighs. The kneeling position is preferred because it provides greater stability as well as isolation of the wrist action.

Kneel in front of an exercise bench which is situated so that the long side is in front of your body. Place your forearms on the bench so that your hands are extended beyond the far side. When you are in position, your hands should be free to move through a full range of flexion and extension. Turn your hands palm down (in pronation) and grip the Strength Bar, barbell, or dumbbells. Keep your elbows bent at 90 degrees so that your shoulders are directly over your elbows or forearms. Keep your forearms in place and lower your hands so that your wrists are maximally flexed (see Photo 10.3).

From this starting position, raise your hands with the weights as high as possible, that is, execute full wrist joint extension–hyperextension. In the ending position, your hands should be almost perpendicular to your forearms, which remain in full contact with the bench at all times (see Photo 10.4). Perform the exercise at a moderate rate of speed and go through the full range of motion. Lower the weights to the original position under control. Pause for a moment and repeat. When using heavy weights or when fatigue begins to set in near the end of a set, inhale and hold your breath as you raise the weights and exhale on the return.

Comments

- To be maximally effective, you should perform reverse wrist curls through a full range of motion. This means that you must move your hands through approximately 100–150 degrees of motion. The exact amount will depend upon your flexibility and the amount of weight you are using. However, if you find that you are moving your hands through only about 45 degrees, then you are using too much weight or have too tight a grip.

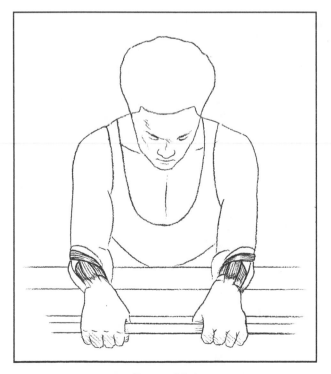

Figure 10.4
Muscles used in the reverse wrist curl

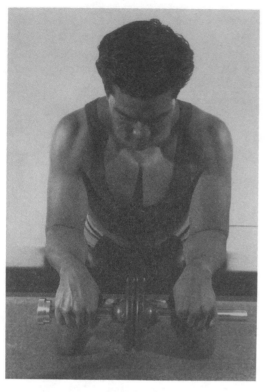

Photo 10.3

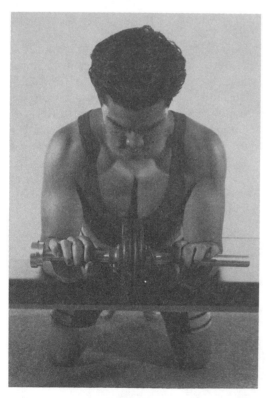

Photo 10.4

• Keep in mind that the heavier the weight, the stronger you must grip it. Because the main finger muscles are located in the forearm, the tendons across the wrist become taut when you lift the weight and do not allow any wrist action. Therefore, use a relaxed grip (as much as possible) while raising and lowering the weights. If you have long fingers or large hands and have difficulty doing the exercise, you should use a two-inch bar such as the two-inch Power Roller bar.

• The extensor carpi radialis longus and brevis and the extensor carpi ulnaris cross both the wrist and elbow joints and have an action at each end. Thus, in order to get a maximal contraction at the wrist, you must keep your elbows firmly stabilized, so be sure to hold them firmly in place on the bench.

• In order to elicit a stronger contraction of the muscles involved, they should be stretched and tensed prior to their contraction. You accomplish this at the wrist when you lower the weights maximally to get maximum flexion. To get stretch and tension in the muscles at the elbow, you should keep your arms flexed at a 90-degree (or less) angle in the elbow joints. This is most easily done if you "lean over" your arms with your upper body during execution. This position also prevents you from involving elbow joint extension (by raising your elbows off the bench) to make it easier to raise the weights.

• It is interesting to note that the muscles most involved are not capable of producing "pure" extension–hyperextension. To do this, there must be helping synergy. In this exercise, the extensor carpi radialis longus and brevis perform both hand abduction (radial flexion) and wrist extension–hyperextension. The extensor carpi ulnaris performs wrist adduction (ulna flexion) in addition to extension–hyperextension. Thus, when these muscles contract, they produce extension–hyperextension, but only when simultaneously neutralizing their tendencies to perform adduction and abduction.

■ Ulna-Radial Flexion

Many bodybuilders and athletes do wrist curls and reverse curls in the belief that they work all the muscles of the forearm maximally, but, in fact, this is not so. Ulna and radial flexion exercises use mostly the same muscles in their other major action. Because of this, for full development of the forearm and to more closely duplicate the exact action used in most hitting activities, you should do ulna and radial flexion.

Major muscles and actions involved

In ulna flexion (hand adduction) the flexor carpi ulnaris and the extensor carpi ulnaris muscles are involved (see Figure 10.5). In this action the little finger side of the hand moves toward the forearm.

In radial flexion (hand abduction), the flexor carpi radialis and the extensor carpi radialis longus and brevis are involved (see Figure 10.6). In this action the thumb side of the hand moves toward the forearm.

Sports uses

Ulna flexion is the key action in the wrist break in baseball and softball batting, the golf hit, the slice tennis serve, and fly casting. It is a key action in frisbee throwing and is used in the racquet sports when you try to impart spin to the ball in the forehand and backhand strokes. In baseball pitching it is used when throwing sinking balls, and in softball pitching it is needed for imparting side spin to the ball.

Radial flexion and the muscles involved are not very important in most sports. However, they are most important in the wrist action in the discus throw and frisbee throw (backhand). Their greatest value is in preliminary movements prior to ulna flexion. This includes cocking the bat in baseball, cocking the wrists in golf, cocking the hand in the tennis serve, and other overhand hits in many other sports. For body-

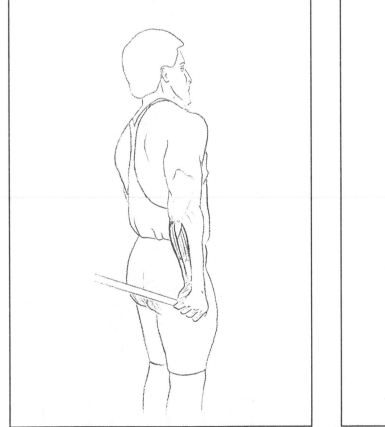

Figure 10.5

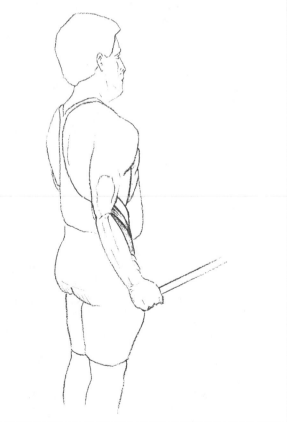

Figure 10.6

161

builders, this exercise is very important for development of the muscles on the inside and outside of the forearm on the thumb side.

Execution

Ulna flexion—Stand up with your feet approximately shoulder-width apart and hold a Strength Bar by the non-weighted end with the weighted end pointing to the rear. Relax your wrist muscles to allow the weighted end to drop to its lowest position, that is, so that your hand is in maximal radial flexion (see Photo 10.5). Keep your arm straight and raise the weighted end of the Strength Bar as high as possible (see Photo 10.6). At the uppermost point you should feel the triceps (long head) undergo contraction. Relax your muscles slightly and return to the original position, keeping the weight under control at all times. If very heavy weights are used or if your muscles get tired near the end of the set, then you should inhale deeply and hold your breath as you raise the weighted end of the bar. Exhale on the return.

Radial flexion—The starting position for radial flexion is the same as for ulna flexion except that you grasp the non-weighted end of the Strength Bar and hold the weighted end of the bar in front of you (see Photo 10.7). Lower the weighted end as far as possible in the beginning position. Keep your arm straight and raise the weighted end of the bar as high as possible (see Photo 10.8). You will note that the range of motion is much less than in ulna flexion. Return the weighted end of the bar under control and repeat. Adjust your breathing when you are fatigued or when the weight becomes very heavy as in ulna flexion.

Comments

- It is important to do these exercises correctly for maximum benefits. The key points are keeping your arm straight, using only your wrist, and raising the weight as high as possible (close to elbow-high in ulna flexion and slightly above the wrist in radial flexion). In radial flexion, avoid a tendency for the biceps to come into play to raise the weight higher.
- Ulna flexion is a classic example of muscle synergy, that is, when muscles work together to allow a specific action to occur. The flexor carpi ulnaris is involved not only in ulna flexion, but in wrist and elbow joint flexion as well. The extensor carpi radialis, which too is in-

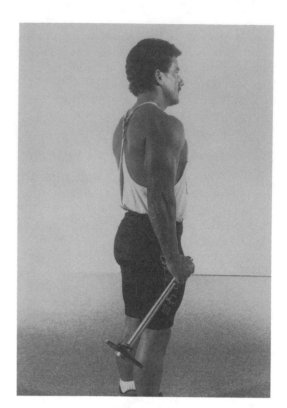

Photo 10.5

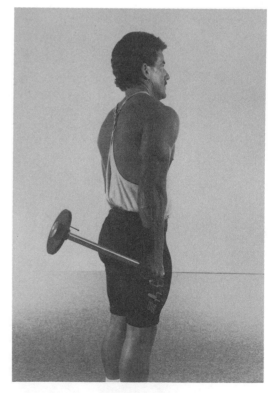

Photo 10.6

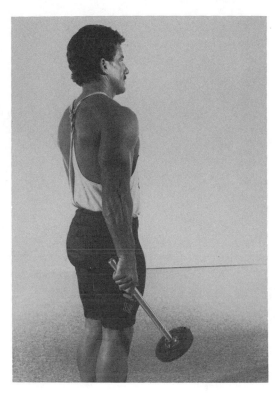

Photo 10.7

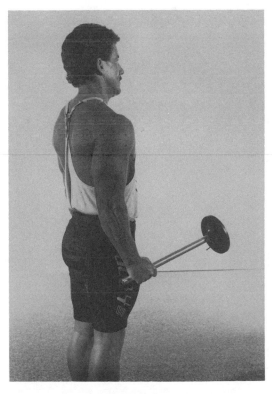

Photo 10.8

volved in ulna flexion, is also involved in wrist and elbow joint extension. Thus, when ulna flexion takes place, the wrist and elbow joint actions neutralize each other and only ulna flexion takes place.

- In this exercise the flexor carpi radialis is involved in radial flexion as well as wrist flexion. The extensor carpi radialis longus and brevis are involved not only in radial flexion, but also in wrist extension. Thus, when radial flexion takes place, the wrist actions (which are opposite one another) neutralize each other's effect and only radial flexion takes place.

- The length of the bar that is used plays an important role in regard to resistance and range of motion. From the practical experiences of bodybuilders and athletes, I have found that the 15-inch length Strength Bar (as depicted in the photographs) is best. When the bar is shorter (8–12 inches), you must use more resistance and the range of motion is less. If the bar is too long (20 or more inches), it becomes too difficult to handle even with the lightest weights. Keep in mind that the longer the bar, the greater the resistance at the end of the bar.

- When using the Strength Bar, it is advisable to start with light weights in order to ensure a full range of motion (approximately 90 degrees in radial flexion and 135 degrees in ulna flexion). Once you are accustomed to going through the full range of motion, you can put additional weight on the end of the bar.

- Because there is relatively little range of motion when doing radial flexion, bodybuilders and athletes have a tendency to do ulna flexion more often than radial flexion. However, development of the radial flexors is very important in maintaining good muscle balance with the ulna flexors. When they are in balance, your chances of getting a wrist injury are greatly diminished.

11 The Fingers and Hand

ANATOMY OF THE FINGERS AND HAND

The fingers and hand make up a very complex anatomical structure. For example, the hand includes 24 bones and over 20 joints. To perform all of the actions at these various joints requires the use of 33 different muscles. The strongest muscles that affect the hand are located in the forearm. These muscles have long tendons that cross the wrist joint and attach onto the fingers or hand. It is interesting to note that these tendons are held together in a very small space at the wrist by a flat band of ligamentous tissue. This is the ligament that is usually cut when a carpal tunnel syndrome operation is done. In addition, there are several small muscles in the hand itself.

Because of the complexity of all of the muscles and actions in the fingers, only some of the major actions that are important in sports and body-building will be described.

BASIC MOVEMENTS IN THE FINGERS

The basic movements of the fingers include flexion, extension, adduction, and abduction. It should be noted that because of the positioning of the thumb, when it flexes, it moves toward the fingers. In isolated finger flexion, the anterior (palm sides) of the fingers move toward one other. In total finger flexion (as in making a fist), the anterior sides of the fingers move toward themselves and toward the palm of the hand.

MAJOR MUSCLES INVOLVED

There are two muscles located in the forearm that flex the fingers. They are the flexor digitorum superficialis and the flexor digitorum profundus. The flexor digitorum superficialis is situated just beneath the flexor carpi radialis and the palmaris longus on the anterior side of the forearm (see Figure 11.1). It originates on the medial epicondyle of the humerus, the coronoid process of the ulna, and the middle half of the anterior surface of the radius. Insertion is by four tendons, which separate after passing the wrist and then go to the four fingers (index, middle, ring, and little fingers). Each tendon splits into two parts at the base of the fingers and then travels upward to insert into the sides of the base of the middle segments of the fingers.

The flexor digitorum profundus is located just beneath the flexor superficialis. It originates on the upper anterior and medial surfaces of the ulna. Insertion is by four tendons, which separate after passing the wrist and then go to the fingers. Each tendon passes through the split in the corresponding flexor digitorum superficialis tendon and is inserted into the palmar surface of the base of the distal phalanx.

There are also three groups of small muscles in the hand itself (see Figure 11.2 for some of these muscles). Their functions are quite varied and they sometimes have more than one action. Because of the extensive detail needed to adequately cover them, they are not presented here.

In regard to flexion of the thumb, only the flexor pollicis longus is located in the forearm. It lies beside the flexor profundus and is attached to the distal phalanx (digit) just as the flexor profundus. It originates on the anterior surface of the middle half of the radius and adjacent parts of the interosseous membrane. Insertion is on the anterior surface of the base of the distal phalanx of the thumb. Other flexors in the hand will not be discussed.

The muscles involved in finger extension–hyperextension, abduction, and adduction will not be described. The finger actions, as important as they are, are not usually considered major exercises in sports and bodybuilding. However, some of the exercises are very important in sports, many occupations, and especially in rehabilitation. Because of this, some of these exercises will be illustrated and explained briefly.

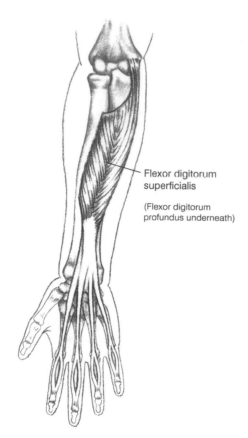

Flexor digitorum superficialis

(Flexor digitorum profundus underneath)

Figure 11.1
Anterior view of the right forearm and hand

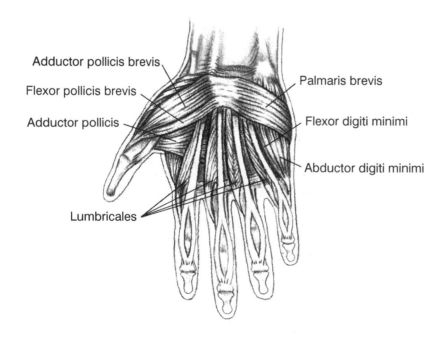

Adductor pollicis brevis

Flexor pollicis brevis

Adductor pollicis

Lumbricales

Palmaris brevis

Flexor digiti minimi

Abductor digiti minimi

Figure 11.2
Anterior view of the right hand

FINGER EXERCISES

■ Exer Ring Finger Flexion

If a survey were taken of bodybuilders asking them what they thought their major weakness was, I feel confident that most would say the biceps or the thighs or the calves. Very few, if any, would say the fingers or the hands. This is understandable because many people take their hands for granted when doing weight training or in their daily work. However, the hands play a critical role in regard to the development of other parts of the body.

The reason for this is your grip, which is the key to how much weight you can lift and how well you perform in sports. The fingers (hands) must be able to hold the weight you wish to use or to withstand the forces created in sports such as football, baseball, tennis, golf, and so on.

Thus, you should work your fingers and hands. The best equipment with which to do this is the Exer Rings (round and flat rings that provide different amounts of tension and resiliency). With them you can duplicate and isolate almost all actions of the fingers. This includes flexion, extension, adduction, and abduction. The best exercise to develop grip is Exer Ring finger flexion.

Major muscles and actions involved

The flexor digitorum superficialis and flexor digitorum profundus are involved in finger flexion (see Figure 11.3). In this action the upper fingers move toward the lower fingers and toward the palm of the hand.

Sports uses

Finger flexion and the muscles involved are very important in all sports that require holding an implement or handling a ball. This includes the sports of baseball, golf, tennis, badminton, squash, racquetball, and hockey, which involve holding some form of bat, club, or racquet to hit a ball or other object. While playing these sports, it is necessary to have a tight grip on the implement on impact to transfer the forces developed by the body to the object being hit. In lacrosse and jai alai, you must catch and throw a ball with specialized implements, and finger flexion is used to control the implement and do this.

In football the hands are used to grip an opponent's jersey or body forcefully, and in boxing the hands must withstand the forces of each blow. Swimmers must hold their hands firm to press against the water to move the body forward. Gymnasts require very strong hands to grasp and hold onto the horizontal and parallel bars and rings when performing. High trapeze artists need very strong grips to grasp a flying

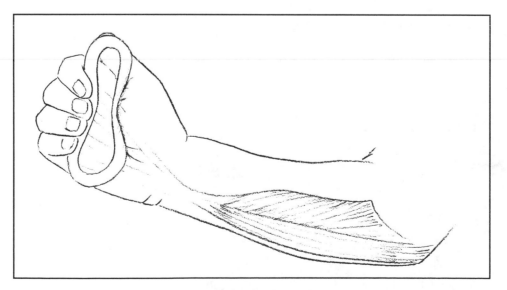

Fig. 11.3
Muscles used in Exer Ring finger flexion

bar to counteract the inertial forces of the flying body. Finger flexion plays an important role in producing force when a football, baseball, or basketball is thrown.

Also, in these (and other) sports, the fingers must be strong to help prevent hitting, jamming, and pushing injuries. For bodybuilders and all athletes who lift weights in their training, finger flexion is very important in grasping and holding the barbell, dumbbell, special equipment, or the handles of any exercise machine. In essence, it can be said that finger flexion (and other finger actions) is needed in almost all sports.

Execution

Select the ring with the needed tension and place it in one of your hands. The ring should be situated against the middle pads of your fingers and the base of your thumb and palm (see Photo 11.1). When you are in position with your elbow bent, squeeze the ring as hard as you can. In the ending position, your hand should be in a fist. The ring at this time should resemble the shape of a paper clip (see Photo 11.2). After strongly contracting your muscles, relax your grip until the ring resumes its round shape and then repeat for the desired number of repetitions. Squeeze and relax in a steady rhythm.

Comments

• It is not necessary to use a ring with maximum tension because it may not allow you to make a tight fist and go through a full range of motion. Going through a short range of motion will not produce the greatest strength, especially grip strength, which is very important for bodybuilders and most athletes.

• Several variants of finger flexion can be done with the different Exer Rings. For example, you can use a ring with less tension (one with a flat surface) by grasping it with your fingertips and then squeezing maximally. This works the joint

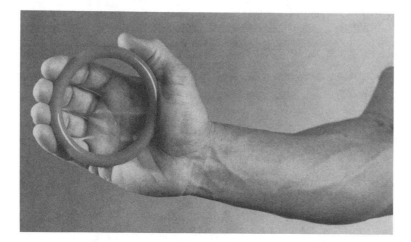

Photo 11.1

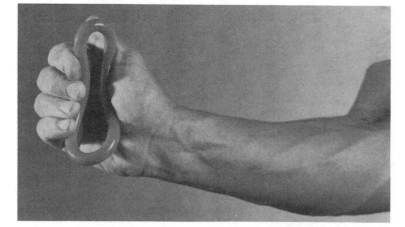

Photo 11.2

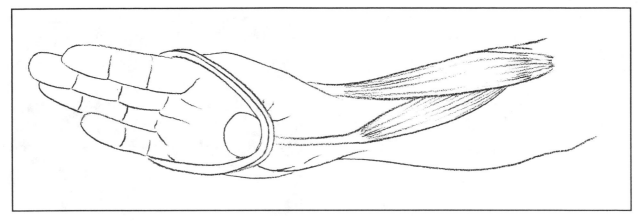

Figure 11.4
Muscles used in Exer Ring finger extension

formed by your fingers and palm (metacarpophalangeal joint). Or you can work one finger individually with a flat-surface weaker tension ring. Place the ring against the upper fingertip or the middle and lower finger pads, and place the opposite "pole" of the ring against your thumb. To work almost the entire finger, hold the appropriate ring in contact with the inner surface of your finger and thumb and then squeeze. In each of these variants, you will notice a slightly different muscle action.

- Finger flexion with the rings can be done in many ways and in many places. For example, you can squeeze the rings while you are standing up with your arm straight or bent at the elbow. If you drive long distances, you can work one hand when it is safe to do so or when you stop at a traffic signal. Some student athletes like to work the rings while sitting in class.

- The rings can also be used in water, and therefore they have great value in rehabilitation. For example, the rings can be used while you are in warm or hot water when your muscles are warm and pliable. This is especially effective for people with arthritis.

- Because some of the major finger flexor muscles are located in the forearm (with their tendons running into the hand and fingers), you will see a definite change in forearm muscle definition after you do finger flexion exercises. In addition, you will develop a much stronger wrist.

- Finger flexion with the Exer Rings is the best exercise for developing grip strength. Other

devices such as spring-loaded grippers do not allow you to go through a great range of motion. The same thing is true with squeezing a tennis ball. And, if you have small hands, you may even have difficulty in gripping these items. Different kinds of putty are also available, but the putty does not return to its original shape after each repetition and must be remolded. Also, putty cannot be used in water and cannot be used for many other finger exercises. The versatility of the Exer Rings also allows for very isolated and specific work of the fingers or finger joints.

OTHER FINGER EXERCISES

■ Exer Ring Finger Extension

In sports and in many everyday activities, finger extension is not important in and of itself. The fingers are rarely used in any forceful extension-type movement. However, finger extensor strength is very important to balance the strength of the flexors and to allow for proper isolation of individual joints of the fingers in flexion. For example, in order to work only the first two joints of the fingers, the extensors must contract statically to hold the bottom digit in place (see Figure 11.4). Thus, isometric contraction of the extensors is very important.

169

Execution

This exercise is executed in three different ways: Place the ring near either the end, the middle, or the base of your fingers and thumb. Extend the fingers in a movement to spread the ring apart and hold for 4–6 seconds. Then relax for a few seconds and repeat. Apply a minimum of 70–80 percent of your maximum strength in the extension movement (see Photo 11.3).

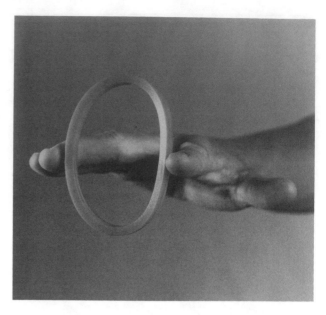

Photo 11.4

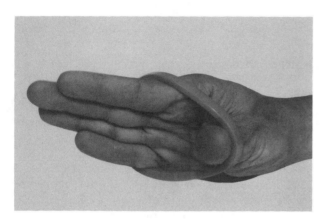

Photo 11.3

■ Finger Adduction and Abduction

These actions are important for musicians, who must have a wide spread of the fingers, and in some sports, for example, in basketball for holding the ball, and in baseball for throwing the fork ball. They are also important in some occupations and in rehabilitation.

To execute finger adduction and abduction, use a flat Exer Ring and place it in between any two fingers fairly close to the upper end of the fingers (see Photo 11.4). When the ring is in position, the tension of the ring will cause your fingers to spread apart. Hold the ring in place with your other hand and then squeeze your fingers together to flatten the ring as much as possible (see Photo 11.5). Relax your muscles to allow the ring to expand and then repeat. Use the heavy-tension flat ring for the stronger fingers and use the lighter ring for the weak fingers.

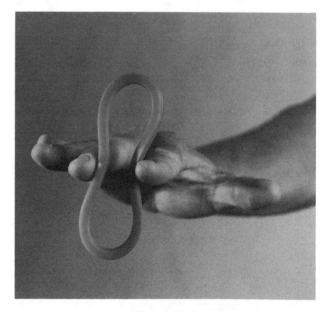

Photo 11.5

■ Strengthening the Thumb

The thumb is very important in some grips and in holding implements. Its key value is in the pinching action necessary to hold something between your fingers and your thumb (see Figure 11.5).

170

To develop this ability, use a flat Exer Ring as follows: Place the backs of your fingers on a flat, hard surface such as a table and then place the ring vertically against your fingers and top pad of your thumb (see Photo 11.6). Hold your fingers in place and use your thumb to depress the ring (see Photo 11.7). If the flat ring does not have sufficient tension, use one of the round rings, but hold it in place with your other hand so that it will not slip out.

The Exer Rings can be used in many other exercises to develop the fingers. These exercises are very important in strengthening the fingers in all of their actions and functions. In addition, because of their value in rehabilitation, it is believed that doing the various exercises, especially flexion and extension, on a regular basis may prevent carpal tunnel syndrome. This problem disables many athletes in the iron sports as well as people in professional and industrial lines of work.

For more information on the Exer Rings, contact Sports Training Inc., P.O. Box 460429, Escondido, CA 92046.

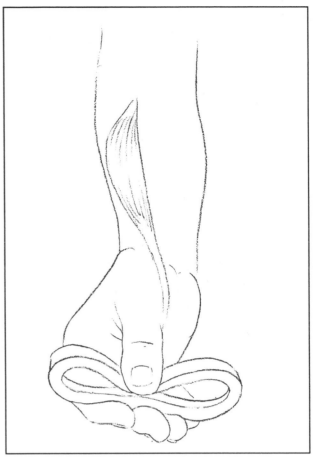

Figure 11.5
Muscles used in strengthening the thumb

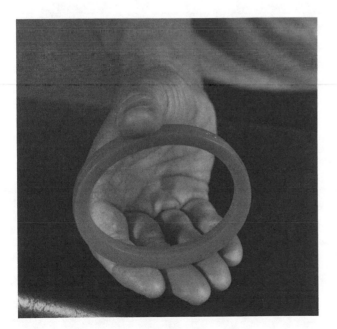

Photo 11.6

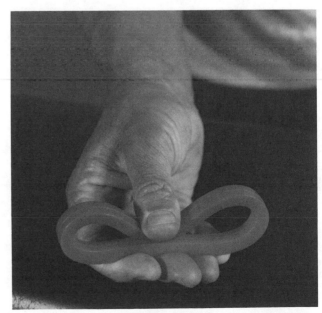

Photo 11.7

12 Combined Shoulder and Arm Exercises

There are many exercises that involve the shoulder joint, shoulder girdle, elbow joint, and sometimes the wrist joint simultaneously or in sequence. These are called compound or multijoint exercises. Examples of these exercises are the bench press, overhead press, dip, pullup, and pushup. However, since many of these exercises overlap each other in regard to muscle involvement, only the more common ones will be described.

■ Bench Press

The bench press is one of the most popular upper body exercises. This is partly due to the fact that it is one of the events in powerlifting and it is important in developing the pectoralis major.

Major muscles and actions involved

The pectoralis major and the anterior deltoid are involved in shoulder joint horizontal flexion (adduction) in the bench press (see Figure 12.1). In this action the arms travel in a plane perpendicular to the trunk. Initially the arms are out to the sides in line with the shoulders and then they move upward until they are above the chest.

The pectoralis minor and serratus anterior are involved in scapula abduction. In this action the scapulae move out to the sides of the rib cage from a position close to the spine. In the elbow

joint the triceps brachii is involved in elbow joint extension. In this action the forearm moves away from the upper arm until the arm is straight.

Sports uses

The actions and muscles involved in the bench press are very important in all sports that require reaching, pushing, or side-arm throwing and striking. Thus, they are needed in gymnastics (push-offs in floor exercises), in boxing (jabbing), in the martial arts (execution of various punches), in football (linemen pushing or hitting with the arms and blocking), in the racquet sports in forehand hits, in the shot put (together with the incline press), in the discus throw, and in other sports. In bodybuilding they are very important for the development of the chest and anterior shoulders, the area under the armpits, and the back of the upper arm.

Execution

Lie on your back on an exercise bench and assume a stable position. For safety the bench should have uprights for positioning of the bar overhead. Place your feet flat on the floor about shoulder-width apart and flex your knees about 90 degrees. Your head, shoulders, and buttocks should rest on the bench, and there should be a normal slight arch in your lumbar spine. When you are set in this position, grasp the barbell from overhead and remove it from the stands (or have it handed to you). Grip the bar with a

173

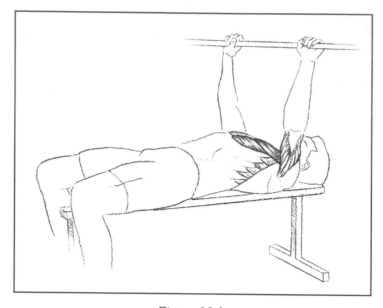

Figure 12.1
Muscles used in the bench press

pronated grip, with your hands slightly wider than shoulder-width apart and your elbows pointed out to the sides. The barbell should be stabilized and should rest comfortably on your extended arms (see Photo 12.1).

When you are ready, inhale slightly more than usual and hold your breath as you lower the barbell at a slow to moderate rate of speed. Keep the bar under control throughout the descent. As the barbell gets close to your chest (see Photo 12.2), quickly reverse directions and push (press) the barbell up back to the initial position. Exhale as soon as you pass the most difficult part of the upward movement to relieve the intrathoracic pressure. Continue the upward movement until your arms are extended and "relax" for a second or two. When you are ready, repeat in the same manner.

Comments

• Starting in the up position and quickly reversing directions in the bottom position makes the exercise more effective. When this is done, the resting inertia of the barbell in the down position is eliminated. More important, doing the exercise this way uses muscle resilience to help get the bar moving upward. It is important to understand that when the bar is being lowered, the muscles involved, especially the pectoralis major and the anterior deltoid, undergo a strong eccentric contraction. This eccentric contraction gets much stronger as the bar reaches chest level. However, if you quickly reverse directions, you can use the stored energy of the eccentric contraction in the upward concentric contraction to give you greater force. But, if you rest in the bottom position, this effect is lost and you will then have to generate additional force to push the bar back up.

• For safety, spotters should always be present when heavy weights are used. They should stand at your sides prepared to grab the ends of the barbell if you need help. It is not uncommon for a bodybuilder or athlete to black out or suddenly collapse when pushing the barbell up and then have the weights come crashing down. If only one spotter is available, the spotter should stand by your head with his hands under the bar during execution.

• Proper breathing can assist you in the lift and can help prevent blackout. When you inhale and hold your breath, your rib cage (chest) stabilizes so that the muscles involved have a firm base upon which to act. But you must forcefully exhale as soon as you pass the difficult phase in the upward push to relieve the intrathoracic pressure as quickly as possible. When very heavy weights are used, you may find it advantageous to release a little air earlier if the pressure is very great. But hold most

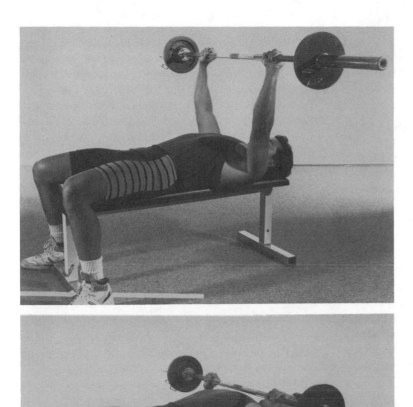

Photo 12.1

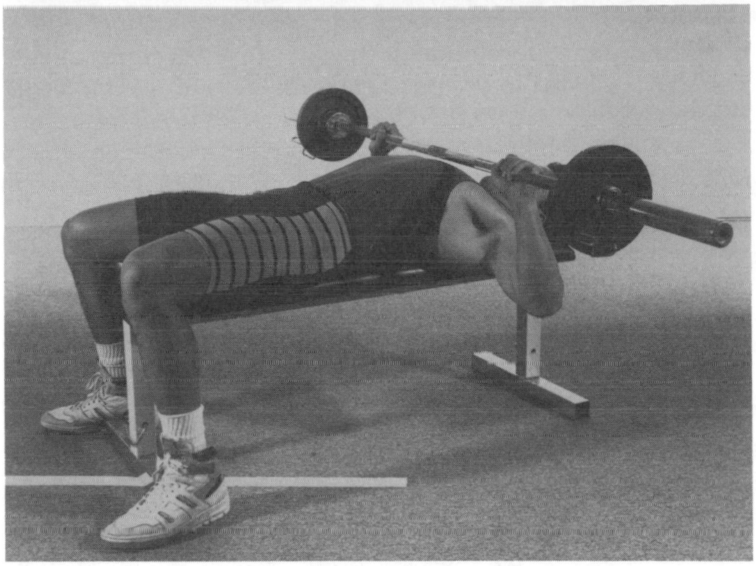

Photo 12.2

of it, as you will need it to complete the lift. Keep in mind that holding your breath allows you to create greater force, and it helps to keep the execution safe.

• Many bodybuilders arch their backs excessively when using very heavy weights. Doing so, however, does not provide for greater development of the muscles involved and can injure the spine. In general, the potentially dangerous excessive arching is the result of forcing the body to seek the involvement of other muscles to raise the bar. In addition, excessive arching changes the execution slightly, and the exercise becomes more of a decline press because of the

raised and angled position of the body. If your lower pecs are stronger than your upper pecs, this may help you get the bar up. More often, this action shows weaker upper pectorals and anterior deltoid. Most effective is to use the correct weights and the muscle rebound effect so that excessive arching does not occur.

• Another potentially dangerous practice is bouncing the weight off the chest to help get it started upward. Doing this can severely injure the sternum and ribs and should be avoided. When you bounce the weight, you must relax your muscles slightly when the bar is in the bottom position. This can be very dangerous!

Also, by bouncing the weight you do not use the resiliency of the muscles to move the weight. Thus, you lose this important muscular development needed in the extreme ranges of motion.

- An effective variant of the bench press is the dumbbell press. In this exercise you hold a dumbbell in each hand and execute the exercise in the same way. However, greater variety is possible when the exercise is executed in this manner. For example, you can execute the press with your elbows in (neutral grip), which stresses the upper pectoralis and anterior deltoid. The lower pectoralis muscles are not involved. Also, with either a neutral or pronated grip, you can get a greater range of motion. For a greater range of motion, reach up as high as possible with one of your arms by tensing more of the inner pecs and the serratus anterior to pull your scapula out to the sides more. In this version you should do each arm alternately.

- The dumbbell fly exercise is also very effective for pectoral development. To perform the exercise, assume a supine position on a bench and hold dumbbells in your hands. Keep your arms straight and in line with your shoulders and lower both arms sideways until they are below the level of your back. Return to the starting position and repeat. This exercise is most effective when it is done with your arms held straight, but be careful not to use great weights (over 20 pounds) because doing so can cause stretch marks at your shoulders.

- The bent-arm dumbbell fly exercise, which is very popular with bodybuilders, uses only the lower pecs because of the lowered elbows. This exercise is not a true substitute for the bench press because the joint action is different.

- The actual pathway of the barbell as it is raised has been a topic of discussion for some time. In general, the barbell takes a slightly curved pathway, but it should end up directly above your chest. The key is not so much where the bar is, but whether the bar is balanced well in the up position. Keep in mind, however, that the more vertical your arms are, the more balance you will have.

- Powerlifters and football players who use this exercise to a great extent often develop shoulder problems, especially when they use very heavy weights. To prevent this, you should do the bench press in various ways; for example, you can keep your elbows in for maximum range and short range, or you can use cambered bars that allow you to go even deeper for greater development of the pectoral and anterior deltoid muscles. In addition, you can use grips of different widths for different effects. For example, if you use a narrow grip, greater stress will fall on the triceps, and a wider than recommended grip will tax the pectoral muscles much more. The use of substitute exercises is also effective.

■ Machine Bench Press

How you execute an exercise is critical to the exact development that you receive, especially in regard to the pectoralis major muscle. This will be illustrated on the Keiser chest press machine, which is also an effective substitute for the bench press.

Major muscles and actions involved

The pectoralis major, the coracobrachialis, and the anterior deltoid are involved in horizontal adduction (see Figure 12.2). In this action the arms move from an out-to-the-sides position to in front of the trunk.

Sports uses

See the bench press for sports uses. Some machines, such as the one by Keiser, allow you to do the exercise unilaterally and in various modes.

Execution

Adjust the height of the seat so that when you are in proper position the hand grips will be approximately at shoulder level. Grasp the handles with a pronated grip and assume an erect seated position with your back against the back support pads. Place your feet on the floor and in front of the foot pedals so that a press of your heel will change the resistance. Before starting, decrease the resistance so that you can fully extend your arms in front of you. This is the beginning and ending position (see Photo 12.3).

When you are ready, inhale and hold your breath as you allow the strong eccentric return to bring the handles into your chest (see Photo 12.4). As soon as you reach this position, quickly

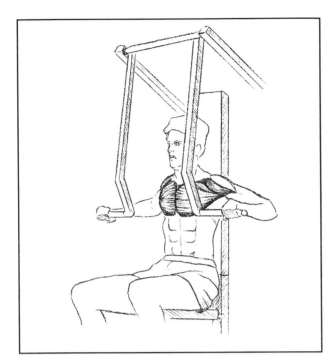

Figure 12.2
Muscles used in the machine bench press

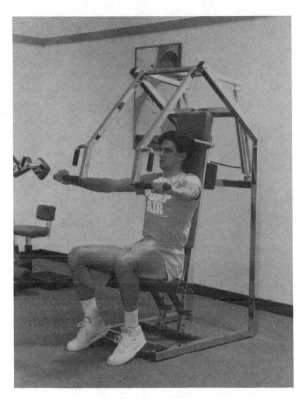

Photo 12.3

reverse without any stopping and push back to the original position. Exhale as you pass the most difficult part of the pushing back movement. Pause momentarily and then repeat.

It is very important that you start with your arms extended in front of you and make quick reversals after bringing your arms back to your chest. When you do this, you use the resilience of the muscles to push the handles back to the original position. If you stop in the back position, you will find that it is much more difficult to push the handles back to the starting position.

Comments

- For variety, the Keiser chest press machine also has a neutral grip. This allows you to work the upper pectoralis and anterior deltoid to a greater degree. Using this neutral grip on a regular basis helps to relieve some of the shoulder stress that builds up from using the barbell with a pronated grip constantly.
- When using the machine unilaterally, you can increase the range of motion. As you push out with one arm, also contract your pectorals more to bring one shoulder forward in protraction, especially when you are using the pronated grip. It becomes more difficult to do this

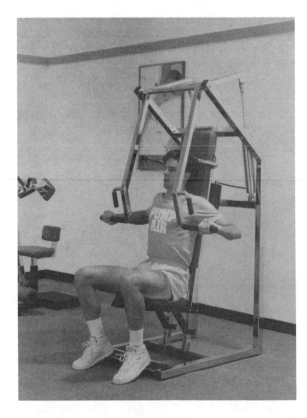

Photo 12.4

if you use the neutral grip. Executing this action allows you to duplicate more closely some of the actions used in different sports such as throwing a punch or a ball or when reaching for a ball.

- When using the Keiser machine, you also have the capability of changing the resistance throughout the range of motion. Thus, you can increase the resistance to do an isometric contraction at the sticking point (the most difficult part of the pushing action), or you can increase the resistance on the return to develop your eccentric strength. It is important to understand that eccentric strength is the key to executing quick reversals from the back position. In essence, your eccentric strength must be strong enough to stop the movement and through the nervous system switch the energy accumulated into the concentric pushing-away contraction. Also, when using the Keiser machine, you can immediately change the resistance if you run into problems when you are doing the exercise.

- One feature that athletes enjoy with the Keiser machine is the ability to do fast repetitions. In this case you must use slightly less resistance and move your arms as quickly as possible through a shortened range of motion. Doing this helps develop faster muscular contractions as well as more speed and explosiveness. Other machines which use weight stacks do not allow such fast movements.

■ Overhead Press

The overhead press was once a part of weightlifting competitions. However, because there was so much cheating associated with the exercise, it was eventually dropped from competition. Nevertheless, the overhead press continues to be a favorite exercise among athletes and bodybuilders. And rightly so, since it is very effective for the shoulders, arms, and overall body stability. There are two main methods of execution: the military press in which the elbows are pointed forward, and the behind-the-neck press in which the elbows are pointed outward.

Major muscles and actions involved

Variant 1—*Military press:* In the shoulder joint the major muscles are the anterior deltoid, the pectoralis major (upper portion), and the coracobrachialis (see Figure 12.3). They are involved in shoulder joint flexion in which the upper arm travels in the anterior-posterior plane from a position alongside the body to the front and upward to an overhead position.

In the shoulder girdle the major muscles are the serratus anterior and the upper and lower fibers of the trapezius. They are involved in upward rotation of the scapulae, in which the right scapula turns counterclockwise and the left scapula turns clockwise when viewed from the rear. In addition, the scapulae are elevated (move directly upward) during execution, which involves the uppermost trapezius and the levator scapulae. In the elbow joint there is extension which involves the triceps brachii. In this action the forearm moves away from the upper arm until the arms straighten.

Variant 2—*Behind-the-neck press:* The shoulder joint muscles involved in this variant are the middle and anterior deltoid and the supraspinatus. They perform shoulder abduction, in which the arm moves from an out-to-the sides

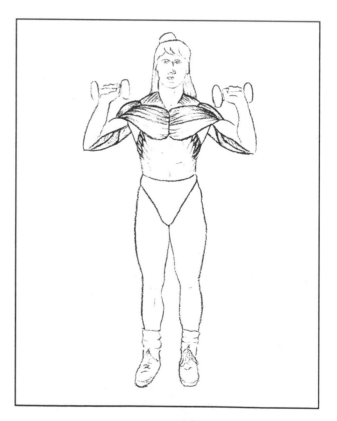

Figure 12.3
Muscles used in the overhead press

position to an overhead position. In the shoulder girdle and elbow joint, the same muscles and actions occur as in Variant 1.

Sports uses

The combination of actions involved in the overhead press is used in a multitude of sports. These actions play a major role in weightlifting (clean and jerk and snatch), in gymnastics (vaulting push off the horse, handstand press), tumbling (pushing off the floor), hand balancing (pushing and holding the top performer), and in the recovery strokes in swimming.

It is used for (but not specific for) all overhead hitting actions, such as the tennis serve and smash, the ceiling shot in racquetball, and the overhead clear in badminton. In basketball it is important for getting the arms up for a rebound, and in volleyball it is important in blocking. Shot putters also find it important for partial development of the muscles involved in their sport.

Bodybuilders use this exercise to build up the deltoids, the area under the armpit (mainly the serratus anterior muscle), and for developing the upper and lower portions of the middle of the back.

Execution

Variant 1—*Military press:* Stand up with your feet parallel and shoulder-width apart. For better balance you can also stand with one foot slightly in front of the other. Grasp a barbell at shoulder level with a pronated grip, with your hands slightly wider than shoulder-width apart. Your elbows should be pointed downward or downward and forward so that in the final position the bar is in front of your upper chest. In addition, the bar should rest on your hands with your wrists slightly hyperextended (see Photo 12.5). When you are ready, inhale and hold your breath as you press the bar upward until your arms are straight and your shoulders elevated (see Photo 12.6). Your wrists should remain hyperextended for better support on the hands. Exhale as you reach the uppermost position, and, when your arms are straight, rest momentarily. When you are ready for the next repetition, inhale and hold your breath as you lower the bar to the initial position and then reverse directions and repeat. Keep the bar under control at all times.

Variant 2—*Behind-the-neck press:* When you are first beginning this exercise, or when greater

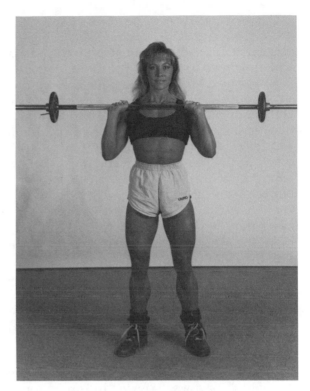

Photo 12.5

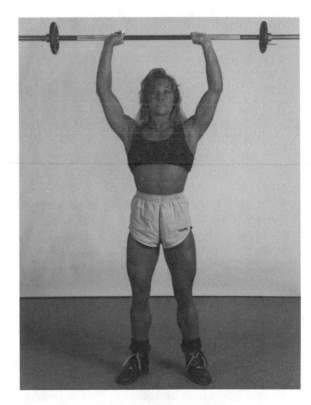

Photo 12.6

safety is needed, execute the behind-the-neck press from a seated position (straddling an exercise bench). Grasp the bar or dumbbells with a palms-down (pronated) grip behind your head (see Photo 12.7). Your hands should be approximately 6–10 inches away from your shoulders on each side; the exact amount will depend on your flexibility. With this positioning, your elbows should be pointed to the sides and downward. The barbell should rest on your hands and, in some cases, on the upper trapezius. With the bar (or dumbbells) in position, keep your elbows back and then inhale slightly more than usual and hold your breath as you raise the weight at a moderate rate of speed. Continue the upward movement, and as your elbows become fully extended, exhale and straighten your arms to rest the bar (or dumbells) on your arms (see Photo 12.8). Inhale again as you lower the bar under control to the initial position and hold your breath as you return to the up position. Keep your back in its normal slightly arched position and look forward or slightly downward during the execution.

Comments

- When you stop in the top and bottom positions, the double breathing pattern used is needed to stabilize your chest so that the required actions in the shoulder girdle and shoulder joint can take place. In addition, this breathing pattern helps you to maintain a rigid midsection, which keeps you from bending your spine during execution and thus helps to prevent injury.
- When executed with the elbows in, this exercise is very similar to the jerk portion of the clean and jerk weightlifting event. In this version, when using very heavy weights, the exercise is done with a slight initial jerk of the arms and a push with the legs (known as the push-press). This action helps to overcome the inertia of the bar and helps to get it moving upward. In this version you stop in the down position.
- When executing the overhead press in a standing position, you must have strong midsection muscles (abdominals, lower erector spinae). They must contract isometrically to hold and maintain your spine in a very firm position. If your spine gives or has movement during the execution of this exercise, injury can result.

- To help prevent the loss of balance when executing this exercise, you should look straight ahead and keep your head in a normal upright position. Looking up may cause you to lose balance and fall backward. Also, looking up places your spine in a hyperextended position and changes the exercise—in this case, you will actually be doing an incline press and if the arching is very severe a bench press! If you are using maximum weights, looking up can cause serious spinal problems.
- Do not think that severe back arching is impossible. In the early days in the sport of weightlifting, when the overhead press was still one of the events, weightlifters leaned backward during execution of this exercise to get a better mechanical advantage to lift the weights. Some arched so much that they actually looked as if they were doing a standing bench press. This severe arching caused many back problems, and because of this the weight belt came into use to prevent the back from becoming excessively arched.
- The overhead press can also be done with dumbbells, especially when a maximum range of motion is needed (see Photos 12.7 and 12.8). If you use dumbbells, you can also do the exercise alternating your arms. To do so, raise your arms alternately as high as possible so that there is maximum flexion (or abduction) in the shoulder joint and also some lateral flexion of the spine. This enables you to reach substantially higher than when both arms are exercised together.
- Another effective variant is to do one repetition with your elbows in front (see Photo 12.9) and the next repetition with your elbows out to the sides as in the behind-the-neck press. Repeat in an alternating manner.

■ Machine Overhead Press

Because of the greater stability required when doing an overhead press in the standing position, many fitness buffs and bodybuilders prefer to do it in a seated position and on an exercise machine.

Major muscles and actions involved

The same as in the behind-the-neck press with the pronated grip in the barbell or dumbbell overhead press (see Figure 12.4).

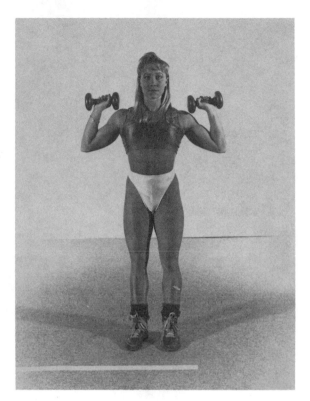

Photo 12.7

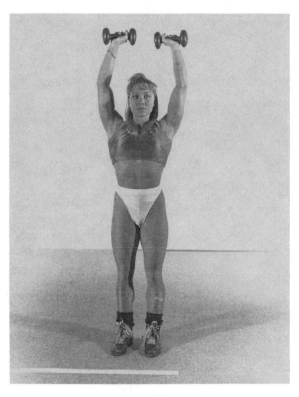

Photo 12.8

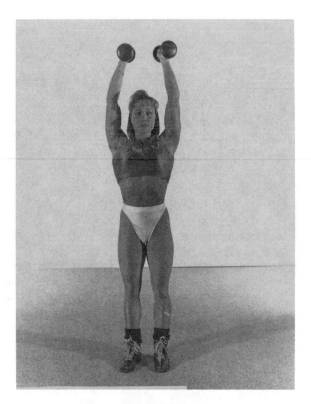

Photo 12.9

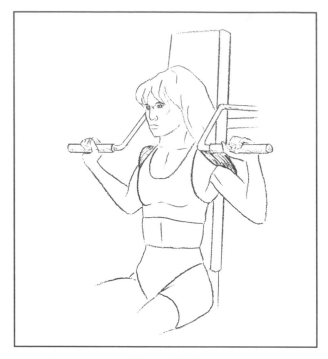

Figure 12.4
Muscles used in the machine overhead press

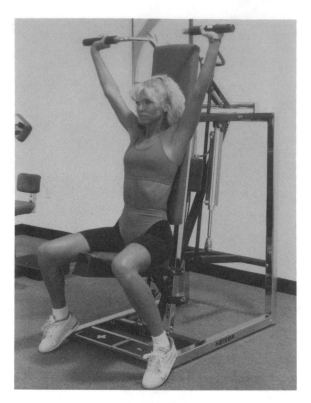

Photo 12.10

Sports uses

The same as for the barbell or dumbbell overhead press.

Execution

Execution on the Keiser overhead press machine will be described, but it is basically the same on other exercise machines. Adjust the seat so that when you are properly seated your hands will be approximately shoulder high and your elbows pointed out to the sides and downward in the ready position. Your feet should be on the floor with your heels close to the foot pedals to change resistance. Your trunk should be erect and leaning against the back support pads. Because the Keiser machine can be used unilaterally, lock the bar in place so that both arms will work simultaneously.

When you are ready, decrease the resistance and extend your arms completely overhead. This is the true beginning position (see Photo 12.10). Adjust the resistance until you feel the necessary tension on your arms. Then inhale and hold your breath and lower your arms until they approach shoulder height (see Photo 12.11). Then quickly reverse the movement and fully extend your

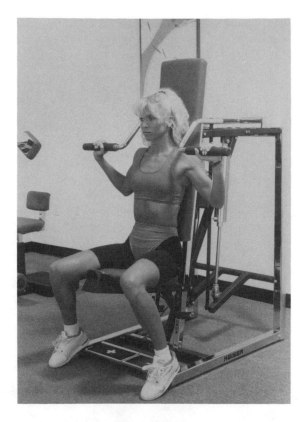

Photo 12.11

arms overhead. Exhale after you pass the most difficult point in the lift in the pushing-up movement. Rest momentarily in the up position and then repeat.

The exercise can also be performed in the following pattern: With your arms alongside your shoulders in the down position, inhale and hold your breath as you fully extend your arms upward and exhale as you return to the down beginning position. Pause in the bottommost position and then repeat.

Comments

- When you start this exercise with your arms extended above you, you can use the resilience of the muscles to reverse directions in the down position. This allows you to use greater force in overcoming the resistance. However, when you use the bottom position as the starting point for the exercise, you cannot use the resilience of the muscles. Because of the great inertia developed in the stationary position, you must concentrate on using your entire body to generate sufficient force to push the weight upward. Beginning in the down position is usually reserved for weightlifters who must do this action in their sport. Athletes, on the other hand, should use the muscle resilience variant because they require greater speed and explosiveness in their actions.
- To assist in developing eccentric strength, increase the resistance on the downward movement, and, when you reach the bottom, decrease the resistance for the return. Also do some isometric work by increasing the resistance at different points in the upward range of motion.
- When using the Keiser machine to exercise one arm at a time, you can also increase the range of motion. As you push up with one arm, elevate your shoulder girdle on that side higher and even laterally flex your spine a bit to enable you to reach even higher. For variety, this can be done with both arms in an alternating manner. These actions are especially important for athletes who must be able to reach as high as possible.
- When doing the overhead press, it is important that you do not max out very often or try for a maximum eccentric return because of the extreme pressure that will then be placed on the spine. When you maintain your arms overhead for a long period of time with great weight, the

compression on the spine is great. Because of this, after doing the overhead press you should always do some stretching activities such as hanging by your hands.

■ Incline and Decline Presses

To further isolate the upper and lower portions of the pectoralis major, you should do the incline (upper) and decline (lower) presses. To do these exercises, you must use an incline board or incline and decline benches for effective execution.

Major muscles and actions involved

Variant 1—*Incline press:* The muscles and actions involved in this exercise are a cross between the bench press and the overhead press. In essence, the movement is diagonal flexion, which uses some of the muscles that are involved in the bench press and the overhead press. Thus, rather than describing these muscles and actions again, just remember that the greater the incline, the closer the exercise approaches the muscles and actions in the overhead press, and the lower the incline, the more the exercise approaches the muscles and actions in the bench press.

Variant 2—*Decline press:* The same concept applies here. In the decline press you do diagonal extension, which is made up of a combination of the bench press and the two versions of the dip.

Sports uses

The same as for the bench press and the overhead press. Note also that the incline press is most important in the shot put, discus, and hammer throw, as it more closely duplicates the specific actions in these sports.

For the decline press, the sports uses are the same as for the dip and the bench press. The decline press is very important in downward pushing actions, which are used in football, swimming (especially the back stroke), water polo, synchronized swimming, flying rings, and basketball. The movements of the incline and decline presses are used in bodybuilding for full development of the pectoralis major.

Execution

Variant 1—*Incline press:* Sit down on an incline bench. Your head, shoulders, and buttocks should be in good alignment, resting on the incline board so that your body is stable. When you are ready, grasp the barbell from above with a pronated grip, with your hands placed slightly wider than shoulder-width apart. Your arms should be fully extended before you begin the exercise (see Photo 12.12).

When you are ready, inhale slightly more than usual and hold your breath as you lower the barbell, keeping it under control. Continue the descent until the bar gets close to your upper chest, at which time you should quickly reverse directions and press the bar upward until your arms are fully extended. Exhale as you pass the most difficult part of the press phase and as your arms become straight. The action should be isolated to your arms and shoulders at all times with strong stabilization of your body, especially your trunk. Rest momentarily in the top position with the bar resting on your arms and then repeat.

Variant 2—*Decline press:* Lie on your back on a decline bench so that your head is lowermost and your feet are firmly secured. Then grasp the bar from overhead and balance it on your arms (see Photo 12.13). When you are ready, inhale slightly more than usual and hold your breath as you lower the bar to your lower chest. When the bar reaches its lowermost position, quickly reverse directions. Press upward until you pass the most difficult part of the lift and then forcefully exhale and fully straighten your arms. Pause momentarily and then repeat. If the blood pressure in your head becomes great, do not perform this variant.

Comments

- If you use a narrower grip and keep your elbows in while executing the incline press, the stress falls fairly equally on the upper pectorals, the anterior deltoid, and the triceps. If you use a wider grip and keep your elbows out during execution, you will stress the upper pectoralis major and anterior deltoid even more. The triceps is less involved. If using these different grips does not feel natural to you, use dumbbells and vary the pathways.
- In execution of the incline and decline presses, you should always use spotters, especially when very heavy weights are used. In the

seated incline and lying decline presses, the spotter should stand behind your head and the bar stands. The spotter should assist in bringing the bar up to the stands and be ready at all times to grab the bar if problems arise.
- To avoid possible injury, you should be careful not to bounce the bar off your chest to assist in the transition from the down phase to the up phase. Bouncing the barbell off the chest can severely injure the rib cage. Moreover, by bouncing the weight, you do not get full use of the muscles to move the weight, and you do not use the muscle "rebound" effect. By quickly switching in the down position, you involve this rebound effect, which allows you to use the energy from the eccentric contraction in the concentric contraction; this makes the movement more efficient and allows you to handle more weight.
- For variety you can do incline and decline presses with dumbbells, which allow you to change the positioning of your hands and thereby ensure the kind of development you are seeking. With a neutral grip, it is much easier to keep your elbows in close to your sides and to keep the movement of your arms in line with your body. With a pronated grip

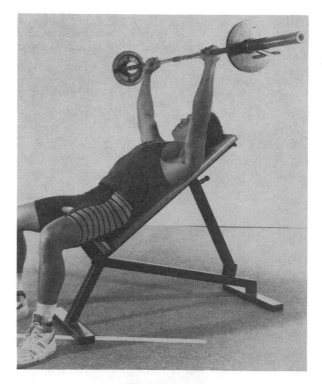

Photo 12.12

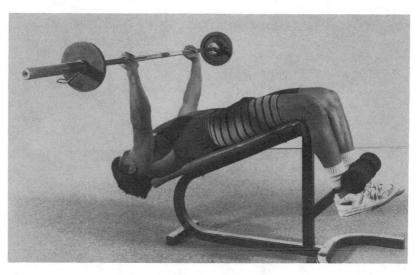

Photo 12.13

and holding your elbows out to the sides, you can stress more of the pectoralis muscle and less of the triceps.

■ Chin-up/Pullup

With the increasing popularity of lat pulldown machines, pullups and chin-ups have been greatly ignored. However, these are excellent exercises that emphasize various muscles. In addition, they can help you to learn to control and move your entire body. Because of this, they should be in your repertoire of exercises, especially if you are an athlete.

Major muscles and actions involved

Variant 1—*Supinated or neutral grip (chin-up):* The muscles and actions are the same as in the narrow grip lat pulldown, but with different stress on the muscles (see Figure 12.5). However, in this exercise the body moves toward the arms rather than vice versa as in the lat pulldown.

Variant 2—*Pronated grip (pullup):* In this exercise the muscles and actions are the same as for the wide pronated grip lat pulldown, but with different stress on the muscles. However, in this exercise too, the body moves toward the arms rather than the arms toward the body as in the lat pulldown.

Sports uses

Chin-ups and pullups include movements that are very important in gymnastics, especially in the pulling-up movements on the horizontal bar, rings, and parallel bars. These exercises also help develop the muscles used in all forms of rowing; football tackling (grabbing and pulling in); all swimming strokes, but mainly the adductor action; all climbing movements, especially rope and mountain climbing; and bodybuilding. Pullups are also very important for good posture because they help keep the shoulders back and produce breadth in the upper back.

Execution

Assume a hanging support position with either a supinated or pronated grip on a horizontal bar. Your arms should be fully extended with your body straight and relaxed (see Photos 12.14 and 12.15). When you are ready, inhale and hold your breath as you pull your body up as far as possible. In the final position your chin should be at least above the level of the bar at completion (see Photos 12.16 and 12.17). Exhale as you lower your body slowly and under control to a full hanging position, pause, and then repeat.

Comments

• For proper execution, it is best to have a bar high enough so that a small jump will be sufficient to enable you to grasp the bar and allow your body to hang freely. If the bar is too low, it will be necessary to bend your lower legs

185

under your body so that you have no contact with the floor.

- When you are using a supinated grip, the biceps brachii muscle has a more favorable straight line of pull, which makes the exercise easier to perform. With a pronated grip, the biceps tendon "wraps around" the radius, and when the muscle contracts, it tends to pull around a corner. Because of this, the load falls on the brachialis and the shoulder muscles. This is why the pronated grip is more difficult to execute.

- It is interesting to note that the major muscles involved (the sternal portion of the pectoralis major, the latissimus dorsi, and the teres major) are the prime movers in either the supinated or pronated grip. However, only the upper latissimus is involved when the pronated grip is used, and only the lower latissimus with the supinated grip. Thus, by using both grips you can get full development of this muscle while still involving the others to almost the same extent.

- When using a neutral grip so that your hand is neither supinated nor pronated, your elbows

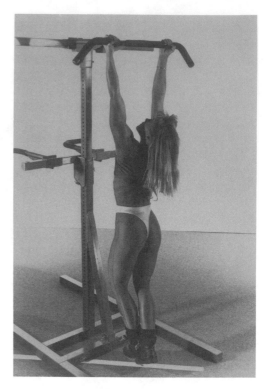

Photo 12.14

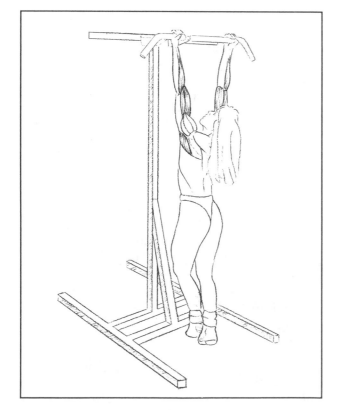

Figure 12.5

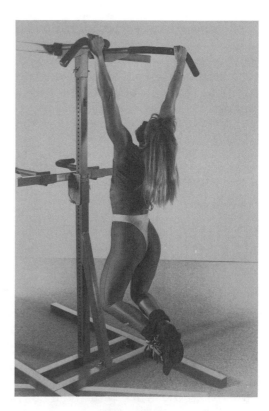

Photo 12.15

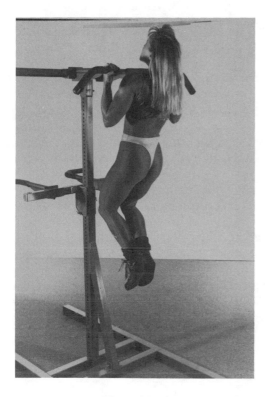

Photo 12.16

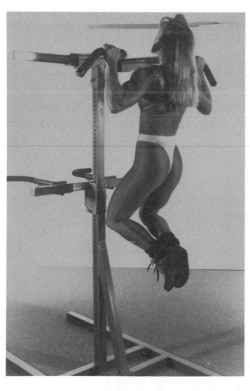

Photo 12.17

stay in line with your body so that the same actions as in the supinated grip occur. However, in this position, the elbow joint flexion may be more effective. The main reason for this is that the brachioradialis has a more favorable angle of pull since there is no tendency to supinate or pronate. Also, the biceps brachii is not twisted in its angle of pull and is very strong in this position.

- The shoulder joint is responsible for initiating upward movement. As the flexion (supinated, neutral grip) or adduction (pronated grip) raises the body, the elbow joint moves into a flexed position. At this time it is more effective to use the elbow flexors in the pull. Also, the contraction of only the biceps, brachialis, and brachioradialis is usually not strong enough to raise a body that is completely extended. Because of its small angle of attachment, the biceps only pulls the upper arm into the lower arm at the beginning of the exercise. (Note that this phenomenon also occurs in the biceps curl exercise.) Therefore, if you are doing pullups or chin-ups for biceps development, you should maintain a slight flexion in your elbows in the down position. However, if you do so constantly, you will lose flexibility and eventually find it difficult to straighten your arms. This, in turn, will limit your triceps development.

- To place greater stress on the upper latissimus, a wider-than-shoulder-width, palms-down grip should be used. The wider the grip, the greater the muscular tension. However, the range of motion is decreased considerably when this is done. When a fairly wide pronated grip is used and the back of the neck is brought up to the bar, the latissimus dorsi muscle pulls in a straighter line and exhibits greater force. The lower pectoralis major, however, is favored when the chin is brought above the bar when you use either the neutral or the supinated grip.

- If you are not capable of doing a full pullup, you should do pullups on a Backmaster machine, which consists of two handles that can be used with the neutral or supinated grip. When using a Backmaster, you can adjust your body position so that you can use your legs to help you do a chin-up. As your arms and shoulders become stronger, you can use your legs less. In time you will be able to perform the exercise with only your arms. The Backmaster is especially valuable for youngsters and the elderly. It can also be used to pull the body upward in a seated position. In addition, using the Backmaster is an excellent way to stretch and obtain low back release, which is most important after heavy workouts, or when you are experiencing low back pain. If a Backmaster is not available, you can do incline pushups, gradually building up to the vertical position. Another alternative is to use exercise machines that counterbalance your weight to make execution easier.

◼ Pushup

Almost everyone has done pushups at one time or another. They are often used as a test for shoulder girdle and arm strength and for setting new records in the *Guinness Book of World Records*. However, how you execute the pushup dictates the type of development that you receive. Thus, be sure you are doing the exercise for the right reasons.

Major muscles and actions involved

Variant 1—*Elbows out:* The anterior deltoid, pectoralis major, and coracobrachialis are involved in horizontal adduction in the shoulder joint (see Figure 12.6). In this action the upper arms move from a position in line with the shoulders to a vertical position under the shoulders. In the shoulder girdle, there is scapula abduction performed by the pectoralis minor and the serratus anterior, while in the elbow joint there is extension performed by the triceps brachii. In scapula abduction the scapulae move out to the sides of the body from a position alongside the spine. In elbow extension the arm straightens as the upper arm moves away from the forearm.

Variant 2—*Elbows in close to the sides:* In the shoulder joint the anterior deltoid and the upper pectoralis major are involved in shoulder joint flexion and upward rotation of the scapula. In this action the right scapula rotates counterclockwise and the left clockwise when viewed from the rear, and at the same time the scapulae move out away from the spine toward the sides of the body. In the elbow joint there is extension, in which the arm straightens as the upper arm moves away from the forearm.

Sports uses

The muscles and actions involved in this exercise are needed in football pushing and repelling, basketball passing, track and field throwing events, boxing, surfing, tennis and racquetball forehand strokes, and gymnastics (especially free exercises). In fact, it is used in all activities that require an extending or pushing action with the arms. For bodybuilders it is especially important for development of the chest, the front of the shoulders, and the rear upper arms. See

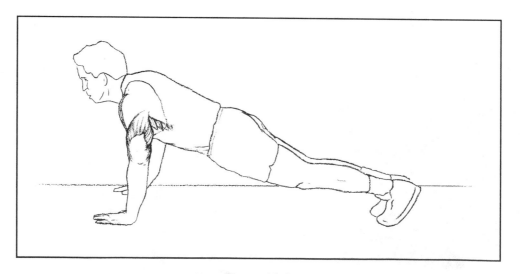

Figure 12.6
Muscles used in the pushup

the bench press and front arm raise for additional sports.

Execution

Assume a prone body position, supporting yourself on your hands and on the balls of your feet. In Variant 1 you place your hands under and alongside your shoulders with your fingers pointing inward toward your body at a 45-degree angle (see Photo 12.18). Your elbows should be out, perpendicular to your trunk. In Variant 2 you place your hands in the same position but with your fingers pointing forward. Your elbows should be in close to the sides of your body.

When you are ready, inhale and hold your breath and make your body firm. Then hold your body rigid and slowly lower it until your chest is very close to the floor (see Photo 12.19), and then reverse directions and raise your body until your arms are again straight. Exhale after you pass the sticking point, or the most difficult point in the range of motion, as you push your body back to the original position. The axis for the movement is in your feet, so you must keep your body rigid at all times during the execution.

Comments

• In Variant 1 it is important for your elbows to remain out to the sides of your body, perpendicular to your trunk. Only in this way will development of the entire pectoralis major muscle occur. When your elbows are held in close to your body, as in Variant 2 (see Photos 12.20 and 12.21), only the upper or clavicular portion of the pectoralis major will be worked. There will also be a greater load placed on the triceps muscle, because only a relatively small portion of the pectoralis major will be in use.

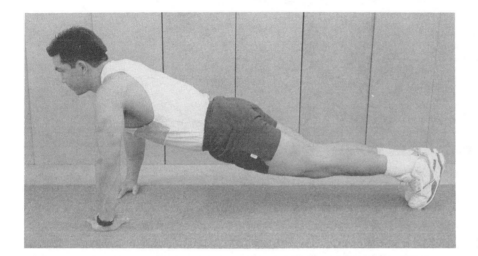

Photo 12.18

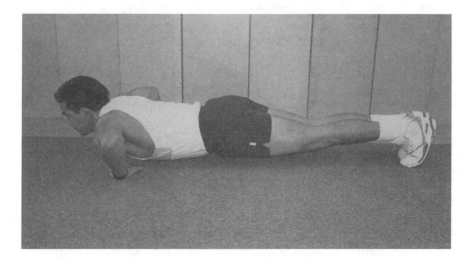

Photo 12.19

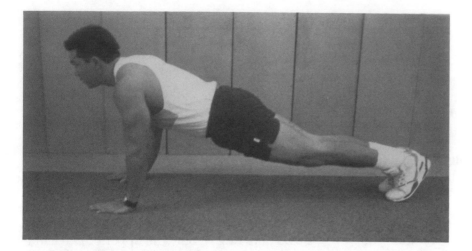

Photo 12.20

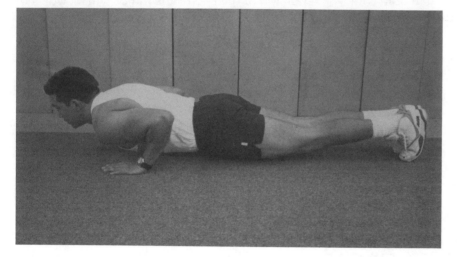

Photo 12.21

When the pushup is done with the elbows out, it, in essence, duplicates the bench press exercise.

• Variations in the placement of your hands have an effect on the amount of stress placed on the muscles involved. If a narrower than shoulder-width placement is used, the triceps muscle will be mostly responsible for raising the body. A wider than shoulder-width placement places a greater load on the chest (shoulder joint) muscles.

• If a greater range is desired in the extreme position, do the exercise by placing your hands and feet on benches or boxes so that your body can drop lower, below the level of your hands and feet. This is an especially valuable variation for total development of the pectoralis major.

• In all variations your body must be kept extended in a straight line from your head to your feet. In so doing, the abdominal and lower back muscles will undergo a static contraction. This, in turn, helps to improve these midsection muscles. However, if you are not capable of doing pushups with your body kept straight, you can do the exercise by supporting yourself on your knees instead of your feet. Make sure to keep your body straight to ensure the correct arm and shoulder joint action.

• To increase the resistance, place your feet on a bench so that they are higher than your hands. This will increase the resistance and change the shoulder joint action only slightly.

■ Bar Dip

The bar dip is one of the best exercises for the chest, back, shoulders, and triceps. Most dip-

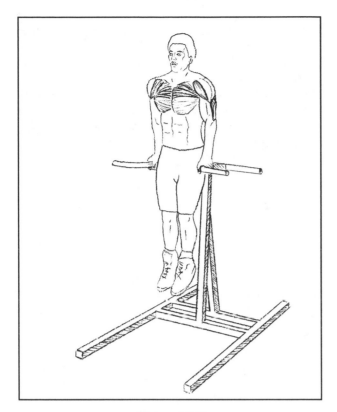

Figure 12.7
Muscles used in the bar dip (neutral grip)

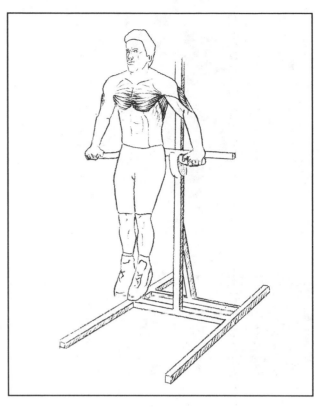

Figure 12.8
Muscles used in the bar dip (pronated grip)

ping bars are similar to gymnastic parallel bars so that when you do the exercise you can use only the neutral grip, that is, with your palms facing your body. But if you want even greater development, you should use bars on which you can also use a pronated grip. This allows for even greater development of the muscles involved as well as other muscles.

Major muscles and actions involved

Variant 1—*Neutral grip:* Flexion occurs in the shoulder joint, which involves the anterior deltoid, the pectoralis major (upper portion), and the coracobrachialis (see Figure 12.7). In this action the upper arm moves from a position behind the trunk to a position alongside the body. In the shoulder girdle the muscles involved are the pectoralis minor and the rhomboid in downward rotation of the scapulae. In addition, the scapulae move downward in a straight line from the pull of the lower trapezius and pectoralis minor. Extension occurs in the elbow joint, in which the upper arm moves up and away

from the forearm as the elbow comes closer to the body.

Variant 2—*Pronated grip:* In the shoulder joint the latissimus dorsi, teres major, and lower pectoralis major are involved in adduction (see Figure 12.8). In this action the upper arm moves in toward the sides of the body from an up and out to the sides position. In the shoulder girdle and elbow joint, the muscles and actions are the same as in Variant 1.

Sports uses

The muscles and actions involved in the dip are needed in many sports which require raising your body when your arms are above your shoulders. They are also used in all sports that require moving your arms up and forward from behind your body or down to your sides from an upward position. Many of these actions are used in gymnastics in the execution of stunts, in free exercise, and on the parallel bars, rings, and other apparatus. The different muscles and actions are also important in diving, basketball, volleyball, and the racquet sports whenever you

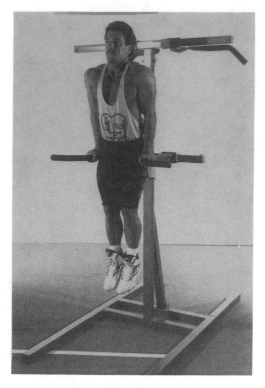

Photo 12.22

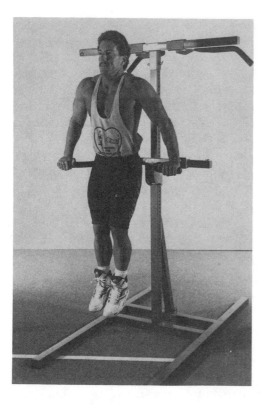

Photo 12.23

bring your arms in front from straight back or from the side rear, in executing various shots, and in blocking and rebounding. The muscles and actions used in pronated grip dips are especially important in all swimming strokes to create a powerful pull and/or push, and in all climbing and other pulling movements.

In addition, the actions and muscles are extremely important to football linemen when blocking or hitting and when pulling an opponent down. They are also used in some underhand throwing actions in bowling, baseball, and softball, for example. For bodybuilders this exercise is especially important in developing the chest, the front of the shoulders, and the upper back and back of the arms.

Execution

Execution is the same, whether you use a neutral grip or a pronated grip. When the bars are in position and at the correct level, grasp the bars using the grip desired and support yourself on the bars, holding your arms straight (see Photos 12.22 and 12.23).

When you are ready, look straight ahead, inhale, and hold your breath as you lower your body by slightly relaxing your shoulder and arm muscles. Lower your body until you feel a stretch in your shoulder joints (see Photo 12.24) and then quickly reverse directions. In the down position with the neutral or supinated grip, your elbows will point to the rear; if you use the pronated grip, your elbows will point to the sides.

Raise your body by strongly contracting your muscles. Keep your elbows and body in place at all times as you push until you return to the initial position. Exhale as you pass the most difficult part of the up phase and as you assume the full, upright position. Pause momentarily and then repeat.

Comments

- If you want to develop greater shoulder flexibility, the exercise can be done with a different movement pattern in which you lower your body and stop in the bottom position and relax. In order to relax, exhale at the bottom while you are holding, and then when you are ready to push yourself back up, inhale and hold your breath as you push to the top position and then exhale. Although this version is more effective for the development of flex-

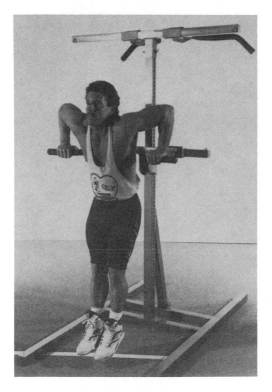

Photo 12.24

skills, but it also helps to prevent injuries which usually occur when the arm is placed in an extreme range of motion under great stress. However, if you find that doing bar dips through a full range of motion is easy, you should hang weights on your waist or hold a dumbbell between your knees for greater resistance. Make sure you still go through a full range of motion with the extra weights.

- The bar dip is used by many athletes for development of flexibility. For example, sprinters who need a full range of motion in the shoulder joints (in the forward-backward movement), use this exercise in the down position. In addition, they do the full exercise with a neutral grip to develop the strength needed to drive the arm forward.

- If you are not capable of doing bar dips through a full range of motion, you should do the exercise in parts. To do this, you will need a small stepladder; you then execute the exercise by grabbing the bars as you stand on different steps of the ladder. Begin by standing one-third of the way down the ladder. Hold for 5–6 seconds and then raise yourself to the upper position. When you can do this easily, use the next lower step on the ladder so that you begin halfway down the ladder. Hold for 5–6 seconds and then push up until your arms are fully extended. After you master this, stand three-fourths of the way down the ladder. Hold for 5–6 seconds and push up. On occasion, go into the full down position and hold it for 5–10 seconds for development of flexibility. Also try to push up so that you get at least an isometric contraction of the muscles in this position. Total movement is not critical in the early developmental stage. By working the muscles in a static (isometric) contraction regime at various points in the full range of motion, you will soon develop sufficient strength to do the entire movement.

ibility, it does make the exercise more difficult to perform. It is easier and more effective to lower your body at a moderate rate of speed and then quickly reverse as soon as you reach the bottom position; this allows the elastic rebound of the muscles to assist you in the return, which is usually quite difficult.

- With a regular (neutral) grip and the bars shoulder-width apart, the triceps is heavily stressed. However, the wider your hands are apart, the more emphasis is placed on your shoulder joint muscles (latissimus dorsi, pectoralis major, and teres major), regardless of grip.

- Extra heavy weights are not recommended for proper execution of the bar dip. The value of this exercise lies in the strength developed in the full range of motion in the shoulder and elbow joints. When very heavy weights are used, you will find yourself decreasing the bottom range of motion. This bottom range of motion is the most important part of this exercise, especially for athletes who need good shoulder joint flexibility and strength. Not only does the bottom range help to enhance various

- If you usually do this exercise with a pronated grip, for variety you should switch and use a supinated grip. This variant uses the same muscles as the neutral grip, but the stress on them is much different. You will find your body moving backward on the descent, which places greater stress on the triceps as well as the upper pectorals and anterior deltoid.

- Using gymnastics parallel bars in various ways can provide you with greater variety in this exercise. For example, you can angle the bars downward at one end and then do the dips on the lower and upper ends. When you do the exercise on the lower end, you place greater stress on your muscles because they must work harder to maintain your body in this position. As a result, your wrist and other midsection muscles will develop to help balance your body during the ascent and descent. When you do the dips on the raised end of the bars, there is a much stronger contraction of the triceps as well as more action in the wrist joint. Thus, for the greatest variety and all-around development of the muscles involved in dips, you should try to use as many different grips and angles as possible.

ABOUT THE AUTHOR

Dr. Michael Yessis received his Ph.D. from the University of Southern California and his B.S. and M.S. from City University of New York. He is president of Sports Training, Inc., a diverse sports and fitness company. Dr. Yessis is also Professor Emeritus at California State University, Fullerton, where he is a multi-sports specialist in biomechanics (technique analysis) and sports conditioning and training.

In his work, Dr. Yessis has developed many unique specialized strength and speed-strength (explosive) training programs. He has served as training and technique consultant to several Olympic and professional sports teams, including the L.A. Rams and L.A. Raiders football clubs, Natadore Diving Team, and the U.S. Men's Volleyball Team. He has also successfully trained many athletes in different sports.

Dr. Yessis has written more than 2,000 articles on fitness and sports training that have appeared in magazines such as *Muscle and Fitness, Shape, Scholastic Coach, Fitness Management,* and the *National Strength and Conditioning Association Journal*. He has also written three books: *Handball; Secrets of Soviet Sports Fitness and Training;* and *Plyometric Training: Achieving Explosive Power in Sports*. He has completed four videos, entitled *Exercise Mastery; Developing a Quarterback's Arm and Strength; Specialized Strength and Explosive Exercises for Baseball;* and *Specialized Strength and Explosive Exercises for Softball*.

FOR MORE INFORMATION

To obtain more information on any of the equipment used in these exercises, please contact Dr. Michael Yessis at P.O. Box 460429, Escondido, California 92046. A bodybuilding video that demonstrates most of the exercises described in this book is also available by contacting Dr. Yessis.